Spanish for EMS

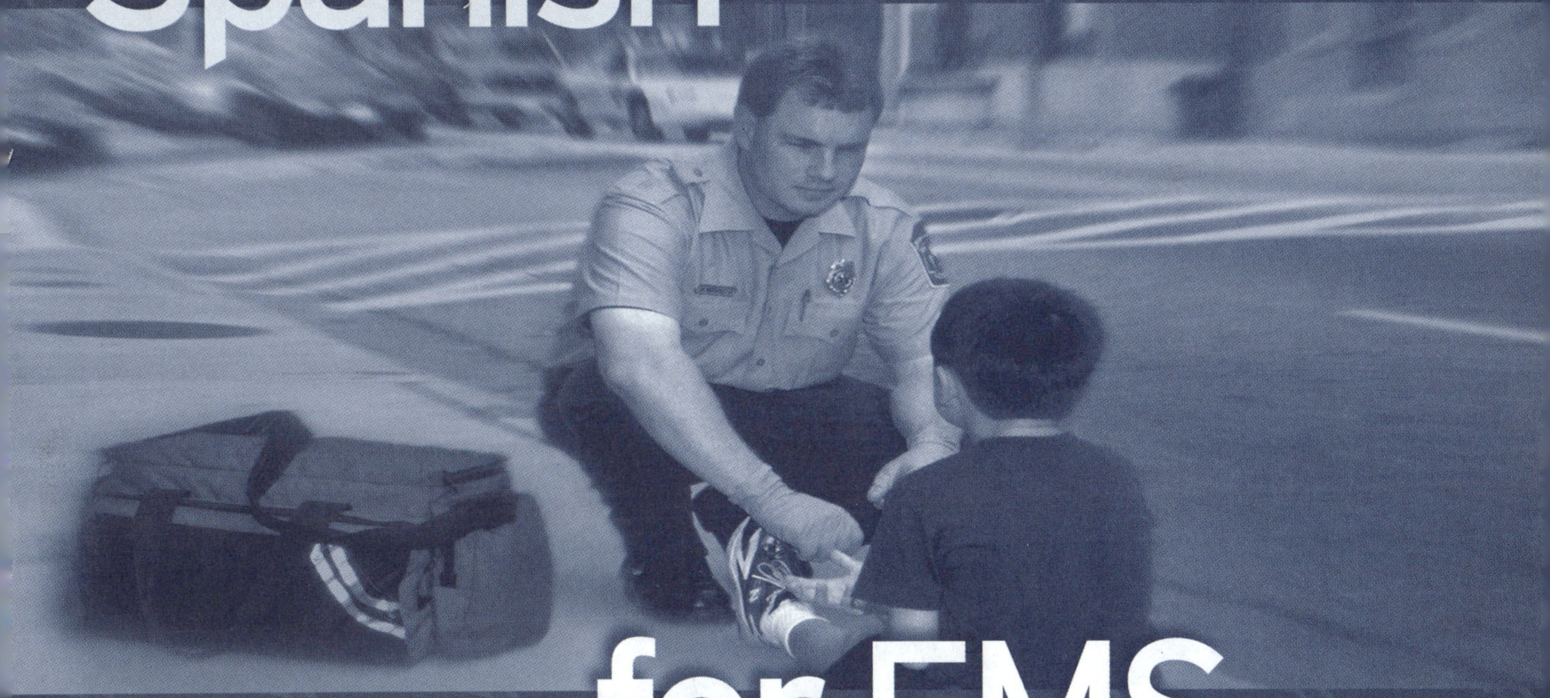

AF777349

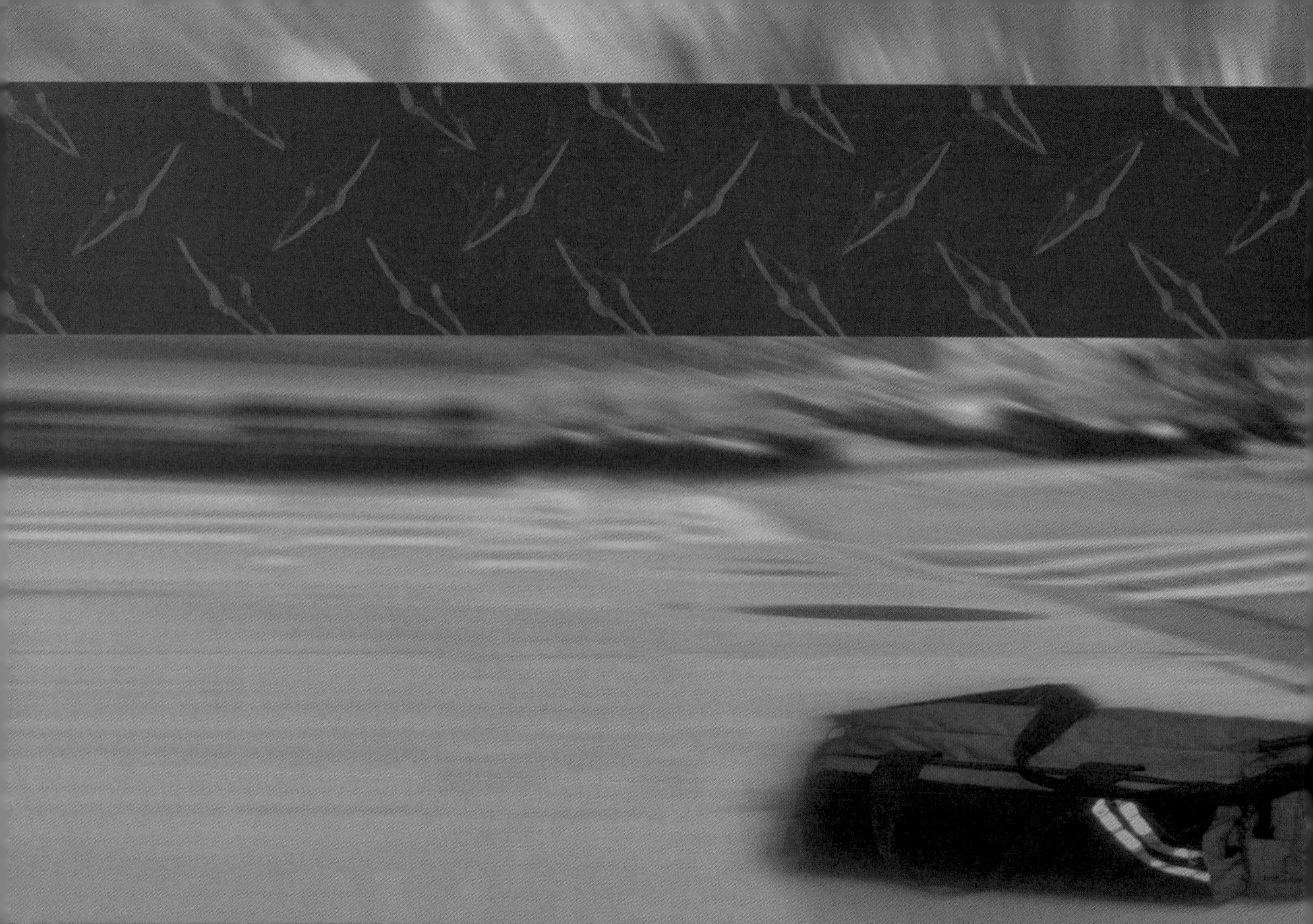

Spanish for EMS

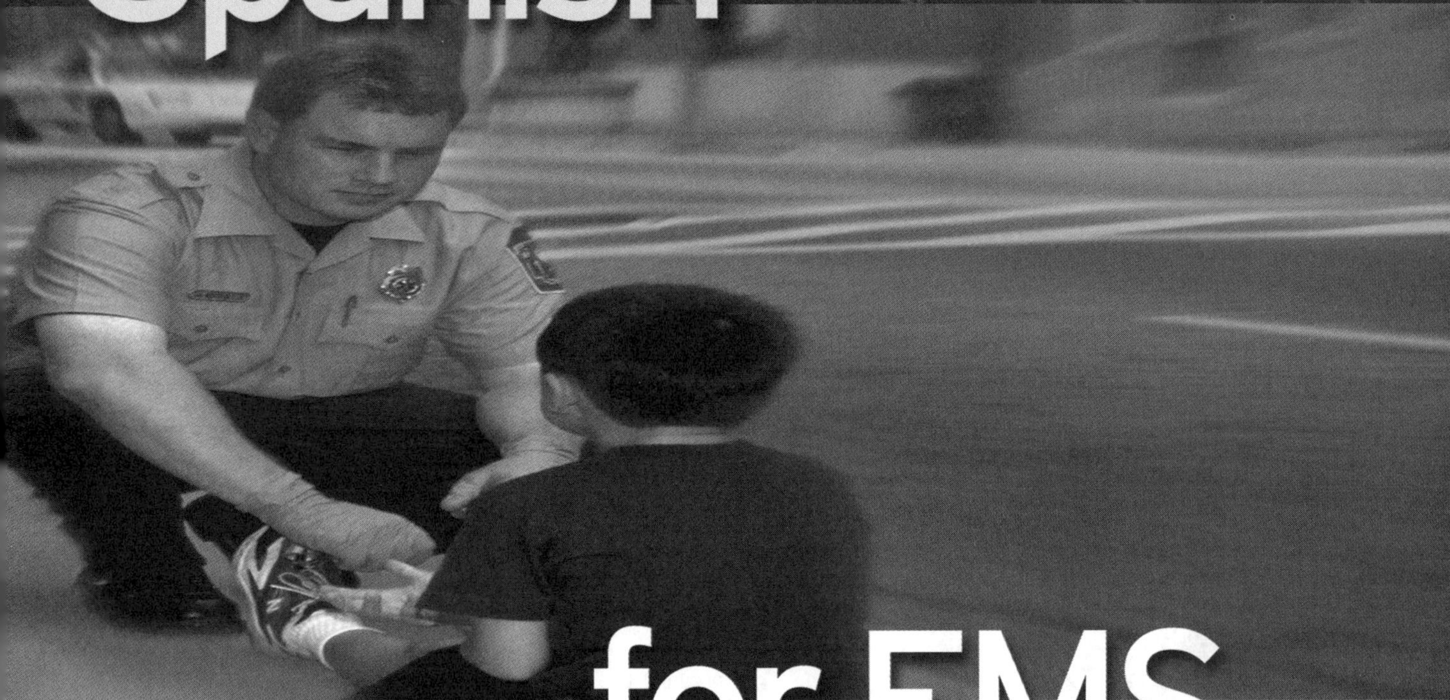

American Academy of Orthopaedic Surgeons

Author:
Aida De La Cruz Dean, MAT
University of Richmond

JONES AND BARTLETT PUBLISHERS
Sudbury, Massachusetts
BOSTON TORONTO LONDON SINGAPORE

Jones and Bartlett Publishers
40 Tall Pine Drive
Sudbury, MA 01776
978-443-5000
info@jbpub.com
www.jbpub.com

Jones and Bartlett Publishers Canada
2406 Nikanna Road
Mississauga, ON L5C 2W6
CANADA

Jones and Bartlett Publishers International
Barb House, Barb Mews
London W6 7PA
UK

Production Credits
Emergency Care Aquisitions Editor: Kimberly Brophy
Associate Editor: Jennifer Reed
Senior Production Editor: Linda DeBruyn
V.P. Manufacturing and Inventory Control: Therese Bräuer
Design and Composition: Nesbitt Graphics
Cover: Nesbitt Graphics
Cover Photograph: © AAOS
Cover Printing: Lehigh Press
Text Printing and Binding: Courier Corporation
CD Production: Dr. Andrew Ross, Universtiy of Richmond

American Academy of Orthopaedic Surgeons

Board of Directors 2001
Richard H. Gelberman, MD, *President*
Vernon T. Tolo, MD
James H. Herndon, MD
E. Anthony Rankin, MD
Andrew J. Weiland, MD
S. Terry Canale, MD
Robert D. D'Ambrosia, MD
Darren L. Johnson, MD
Thomas P. Sculco, MD
James N. Weinstein, MD
David A. Halsey, MD
Lowry Jones, Jr, MD
Maureen Finnegan, MD
Gary E. Friedlaender, MD
Peter C. Amadio, MD
William W. Tipton, Jr, MD *(ex officio)*

Editorial Credits
Vice President, Education Programs: Mark W. Wieting
Director of Publications: Marilyn L. Fox, PhD
Managing Editor: Lynne Roby Shindoll
Senior Editor: Barbara A. Scotese

Copyright © 2002 by Jones and Bartlett Publishers, Inc.

All rights reserved. No part of the material protected by this copyright notice may be reproduced or utilized in any form, electronic or mechanical, including photocopying, recording, or by any information storage and retrieval system, without written permission from the copyright owner.

The procedures and protocols in this book are based on the most current recommedations of responsible medical sources. The American Academy of Orthopaedic Surgeons and the publisher, however, make no guarantee as to, and assume no responsibility for the correctness, sufficiency or completeness of such information or recommendations. Other or additional safety measures may be required under particular circumstances.

This textbook is intended solely as a guide to the appropriate procedures to be employed when rendering emergency care to the sick and injured. It is not intended a statement of the standards of care required in any particular situation, because circumstances and the patient's physical condition can vary widely from one emergency to another. Nor is it intended that this textbook shall in any way advise emergency personnel concerning legal authority to perform the activities or procedures discussed. Such local determinations should be made only with the aid of legal counsel.

Library of Congress Cataloging-in-Publication Data

Dean, Aida.
Spanish for EMS / Aida Dean; American Academy of Orthopaedic Surgeons.
p. cm.
English and Spanish.
ISBN 0-7637-2069-0
1. Spanish language—Conversation and phrase books (for medical personnel) 2. Spanish language—I. American Academy of Orthopaedic Surgeons. II. Title

PC4120.M3 D43 2002
468.3'421'02461—dc21

2001058184

Additional credits appear on page viii, which constitutes a continuation of the copyright page.

Printed in the United States of America
06 05 04 03 02 10 9 8 7 6 5 4 3 2 1

Contents

Walk-Through

Spanish for EMS is a self-teaching Spanish course, composed of a book and a CD, designed with the EMS provider in mind. It offers you access to quick and easy phrases and questions in Spanish for those situations where English will not suffice. After completing this course, you will be able to obtain the necessary information from the patient, while defusing a chaotic scene. The course is based on oral and listening practice and it is essential that you listen and speak throughout. It is also important that you visualize situations where you might use the phrases and questions as they are presented. Language is easier to learn if it becomes relevant to you. Remember that learning to speak another language is a lot like learning a skill. It requires practice and commitment. ¡Buena suerte! (Good luck!)

Preliminary Lessons

The course starts with two preliminary lessons. They are designed to give you an overview of what is to come throughout the course. Whatever you do, do not get bogged down here.

Chapter Lessons

There are eight chapter lessons that provide you with vocabulary and examples of the word's usage and practice. Here is how the chapters are organized.

I. Vocabulary 1

AUDIO CD

Listen and repeat the phrases and words below. The longer phrases have been divided into more manageable groupings. Also, practice the first seven phrases until you are comfortable with them before moving on to the next six. All of these will be repeated throughout the book/program so don't worry if you don't memorize them immediately but do become familiar with pronouncing them. Remember that short, frequent daily practice is better than one long practice several days apart.

Commands	
Cálmese.	Calm down.
Silencio, por favor.	Silence, please.
Siéntese.	Sit down.
No se preocupe.	Don't worry.

II. Dialogue

AUDIO CD

You will hear/read a series of dialogues in which you have arrived at a scene and have determined that no one will be able to translate for you.

You arrive at the scene of an auto accident.

EMT	**Señor, ¿habla inglés?**
Patient	**No, sólo hablo español.**
EMT	**Hablo un poco de español.**
Patient	**¡Ay! Estoy muy adolorido. Ayúdeme, por favor (patient talks too fast).**
EMT	**Por favor, no comprendo. Tengo unas preguntas.** *(Here the paramedic begins to ask his questions.)*
Translation	
EMT	**Sir, do you speak English?**
Patient	**No, I don't speak English.**

I. Vocabulary 1: The basic vocabulary you need is presented and a short practice is provided. You should concentrate on listening for recognition and begin to visualize yourself using the phrases and questions. Extensive practice is not needed at this point.

II. Dialogues: These dialogues are designed to allow you to read and hear how the phrases and questions might be used in a real life situation. A translation in English is also provided so you can follow the conversations easily and without frustration. You should listen several times to each dialogue while reading it until you feel comfortable. You may want to repeat after the "EMT" speaker, in order to practice the phrases and questions, but only listen to the responses given by the "patient." You will gain a great deal by listening to the dialogue each time you work on a particular chapter. It trains the ear and will make learning Spanish easier.

III. Practice

Write and say in English the translations of the following Spanish phrases. Remember that you may do the exercise as often as it is necessary to become comfortable with it. Don't limit yourself to practicing it only once.

1. Silencio, por favor.
2. Tengo unas preguntas.
3. Más despacio.

IV. Vocabulary 2

The following are phrases and words that were presented in the earlier dialogues that you might hear at the scene. Listen and read these phrases so that you may become familiar with them. Memorization is not necessary but it is a good idea to have an idea of what the patients may be saying.

Ayuda	Help
Ayúdeme	Help me
Dolor	Pain
iQué dolor!	It hurts! (How it hurts!)
Está sangrando.	He/she is/ you are bleeding.
Está vomitando.	He/she is/ you are vomiting.

V. Review

Go back and listen again to the dialogue. How well are you able to understand what the people are saying? You should notice that you understand quite a bit now. Great job! Think of what phrases and questions will be helpful to you from this chapter. Write them down on cards and begin keeping a file of them in order to review them daily. You're now ready to move on to the next chapter.

VI. Cultural Capsule

Hispanics and Latinos in the United States

Today there are 25 to 30 million Hispanics and Latinos living in the United States, and Spanish is the second most spoken language. Many Hispanics and Latinos have become "Americanized" but others, especially the elderly or newly emigrated, still cling to their heritage and language. In many cities there are pockets of "Spanish only" sections where Hispanics are able to live without ever using English as they go about their daily affairs. While many immigrants are thankful for being in the United States, some find it difficult to embrace a new culture that is so very different from that of their native country.

The terms "Hispanic" and "Latino" encompass a large group of people who are from different countries, cultures, and backgrounds. Although there are similarities due to a common language and historical background, it is a mistake to try to fit all Hispanics and Latinos into one mold.

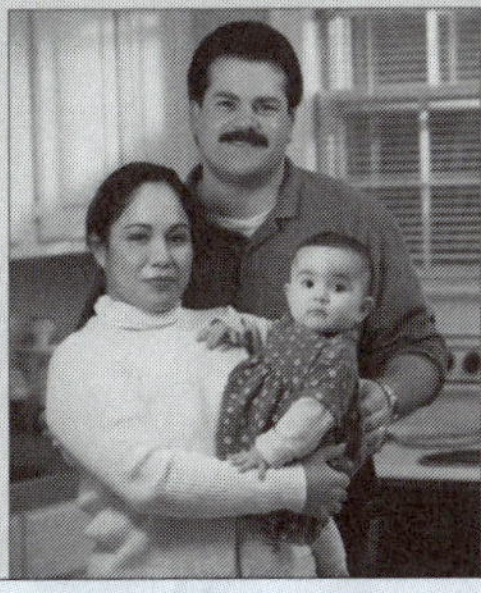

III. Practice: The practices are designed to give you plenty of opportunities to use the phrases and questions presented in the dialogue. There are several different types of exercises, but they have all been designed to help you recall the material, not merely recognize it. However, since recalling material is so much more difficult than recognizing it, a key to memorization is to tie the material to something that is relevant to you. A good way to do this is by visualizing yourself using the Spanish phrases and questions at a scene. Remember, spend as much time as you wish on each exercise, but quit as soon as you feel you are overloading. Your brain can only take so much of a foreign language!

IV. Vocabulary 2: In this section you will find the phrases used by the patients in the chapter dialogue. Although some practice is given, the emphasis is more on recognition than on recall. At a scene it is a relief to be able to understand a little of what is being said, but a lengthy conversation is not needed. Therefore, listen and try to understand the speakers but, unless you are really committed, there is little need to memorize the phrases.

V. Review: In this section you will be asked to review the material and put it all together.

VI. Seven **Cultural Capsules** have been included which present some ethnic differences that may be relevant in emergency situations.

Appendices

There are several appendices included:

- Appendix A lists not only the main questions and phrases that have appeared throughout the course, but a few new ones that may be helpful.
- Appendix B presents vocabulary for some of the more common illnesses.
- Appendix C has a list of the more colloquial expressions for certain body parts.
- Appendix D deals with numbers and time.
- Appendix E has the Spanish vocabulary for family members.
- Appendix F has a sample bilingual insurance form that you may need to fill out for the patient.
- Appendix G contains an Equipment List in English and Spanish.

Answers

Written answers to all of the exercises are given at the end of the book.

Audio CD Icon

The audio CD icon indicates where you will need to listen to the audio CD and follow along in the book.

Acknowledgments

Jones and Bartlett Publishers and the author would like to thank the following people for reviewing this course:

Jose Salazar, MPH, NREMT-P
Loudon County Fire and Rescue
Leesburg, VA

Jonathan Woolery, MPH, NREMT-P, CHES
Medic One Medical Services
Grand Terrace, CA

Author Dedication

The author would like to thank the following people for their support and encouragement:

Her husband, Stephen Dean
Her parents, Roberto and Aida de la Cruz
Her children, Alicia and Michael
Mike Taigman
Jennifer Reed

Photo Credits

Interior photos for this text have been provided by the American Academy of Orthopaedic Surgeons unless otherwise indicated below.

Chapter 1

Cultural Capsule © 2001 Thinkstock LLC

Chapter 2

Figure 2.1 © PhotoDisc;
Cultural Capsule © 2001 Thinkstock LLC

Chapter 3

Figure 3.1 © PhotoDisc

Chapter 4

Cultural Capsule © 2001 Thinkstock LLC

Chapter 5

Cultural Capsule © PhotoDisc

Chapter 7

Cultural Capsule © 2001 Thinkstock LLC

Preliminary Lesson 1

A Guide to Pronunciation

The pronunciation of a second language comes with ease when we are children but becomes more difficult as our native language becomes ingrained and we become accustomed to one set of sounds. In studying another language, we notice that although the letters may look alike, the sounds vary from language to language. We must train ourselves again in understanding and pronouncing different sounds. Below you will find a brief guide to the Spanish pronunciation of the vowels and of some consonants that may be difficult for the English speaker.

Before we begin with the sounds, you should know that accents are a natural part of the Spanish language. Usually the accent designates which syllable is stressed. However, accents are also used to differentiate between certain words that are spelled the same (tu=your, tú=you) and are always used on interrogatory words (¿qué? = what?).

AUDIO CD

I. Vowels: The sounds are constant and clear at all times. Never "shwa" a vowel.

A = "ah" (like in father)
para casa

E = "eh" (like in feather)
bebé este te

I = "ee" (like in fee, "y" acts as a vowel at times and is pronounced like "i")
mi sí soy voy

O = "o" (like in for; be sure not to glide it)
como poco

U= "oo" (like in boo, or the "ue" in Sue)
su un

II. Combination of vowels: At times, two vowels occur together and, although both sounds are pronounced, they run together and become one syllable.

quién siéntese cuándo

III. Consonants: Below is a list of seven difficult consonants in Spanish that may confuse the English speaker.

C The Spanish "c" has two distinct sounds. The "c" is pronounced like "k" or like an "s" (in Latin America).

The "k" sound occurs when followed by "a, o, u," "r" and "l."

camilla casa cruz claro

The "s" sound occurs when followed by "e" and "i."

ciudad policía

G The Spanish "g" also has two sounds. The "g" is pronounced like the English "h" in "he" or like the "g" in "go." The English "g" sound in "gentle" does **not** occur with the Spanish "g." This is a common error for English speakers.

The "h" sound occurs when followed by "e" or "i."

gente gimnasio

The "go" sound occurs when followed by "a, o, u" and consonants.

gota gato

In the combinations of "gue" and "gui", the "u" is silent and the "g" sounds like the "g" in "go."

guía alguien

Q The Spanish "q" is used in the combinations of "que" or "qui." The "q" is pronounced like a "k" and the "u" is always silent.

qué quién

J The "j" is pronounced like the English "h."

julio juego

Y and LL Both of these are pronounced like the "y" in "yes."

llamo yo

H The Spanish "h" is always silent.

hablo hola

ñ The "ñ" is pronounced with a nasal tone. It is similar to the "n" in "onion" or the "ny" in "canyon."

niño señor

Preliminary Lesson 2

The Body

Below you will find a diagram of a body in which the parts have been labeled in Spanish. Also you will note that the question "Does ________ hurt?" has been translated in Spanish for you and a brief practice session given. As you work with this question, keep in mind that it has been translated for *meaning* instead of literally. Spanish does not employ the helping verbs "does" or "did" in order to form questions. Literally the question, "¿Le duele ________?" translates to "To you hurts ________?". This explanation is not to confuse you but to help you in forming questions of your own once you feel more confident.

Question: ¿Le duele ________? — Does ________ hurt?

Example: ¿Le duele el brazo? — Does your arm hurt?

(Notice that in Spanish the articles for *"the,"* which are "el" or "la," may be used instead of the possessive "su" *"your;"* however, you may always use "su" if you wish.)

la cabeza	the head
el cuello	the neck
la garganta	the throat

el ojo	the eye
el oído	the inner ear
la nariz	the nose
la boca	the mouth

los hombros	the shoulders
el brazo	the arm
la mano	the hand
los dedos	the fingers

el pecho	the chest
el corazón	the heart
los pulmones	the lungs
el estómago	the stomach
el abdomen	the abdomen
el pélvis	the pelvis

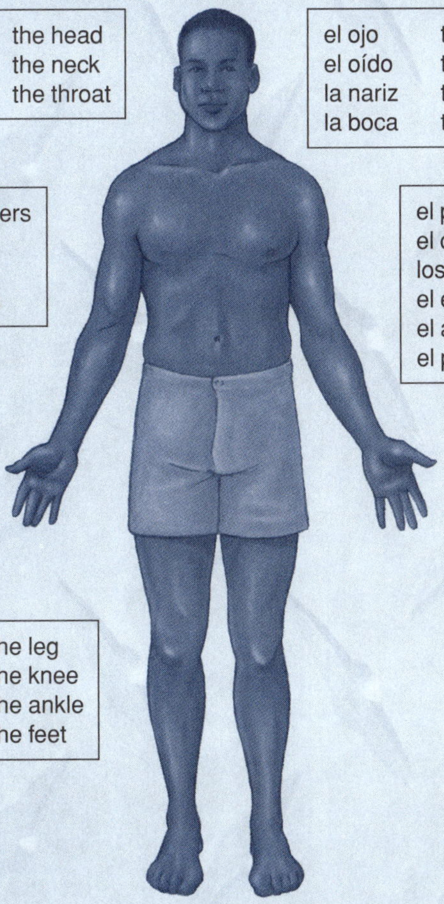

la pierna	the leg
la rodilla	the knee
el tobillo	the ankle
los pies	the feet

Practice

1. Listen and repeat the questions after the speaker. You will hear a response for each question. You may also repeat the answer that the patient gives. We will be going through the whole body and you may look at the picture as you listen and repeat.

   Example: *You:* ¿Le duele la cabeza? *Patient:* Sí, me duele la cabeza.

2. Now you will ask the question "¿Le duele ________?" after being given the question in English.

   Example: *Speaker:* Does your arm hurt? *You:* ¿Le duele el brazo?

Chapter 1

Arrival at the Scene

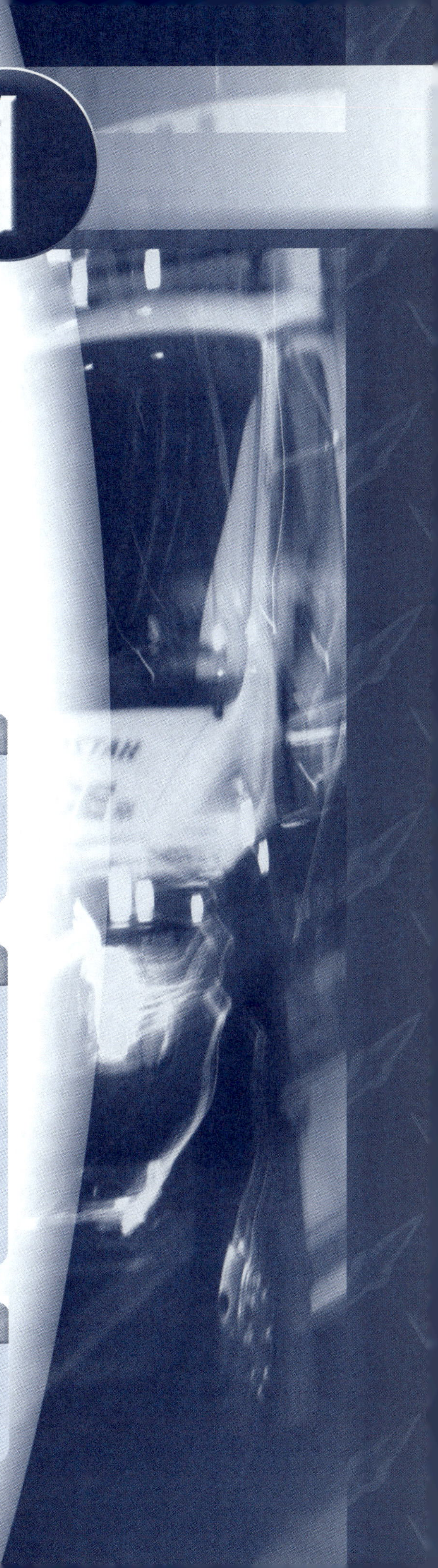

I. Vocabulary 1

AUDIO CD

Listen and repeat the phrases and words below. The longer phrases have been divided into more manageable groupings. Also, practice the first seven phrases until you are comfortable with them before moving on to the next six. All of these will be repeated throughout the book so don't worry if you don't memorize them immediately but do become familiar with pronouncing them. Remember that short, frequent daily practice is better than one long practice every few days.

Commands

Cálmese.	Calm down.
Silencio, por favor.	Silence, please.
Siéntese.	Sit down.
No se preocupe.	Don't worry.

Statements

Hablo español.	I speak Spanish.
Más despacio.	Slower.
No comprendo.	I don't understand.
Necesito examinarlo(la).*	I need to examine you.
Tengo unas preguntas.	I have some questions.
*Vamos a ayudar.	We're going to help you.

** "Lo" and "la" are direct object pronouns meaning "you," "him," or "her" (lo = masculine, la = feminine).*

Questions

¿Es usted el paciente?	Are you the patient?
¿Quién necesita ayuda?	Who needs help?
¿Le duele mucho o poco?	Does it hurt a lot or a little?

Now, you will be given a situation in which you will need to use one or more of the above phrases. Read the situation and choose the best response from the answers provided. You may find that more than one answer may be possible.

1. There are children present and they are crying.
   a. Silencio, por favor.
   b. No se preocupe.
   c. Vamos a ayudar.
2. Several people are involved in an auto accident.
   a. Más despacio.
   b. ¿Quién necesita ayuda?
   c. Vamos a ayudar.
3. The patient is speaking very rapidly.
   a. Más despacio.
   b. Vamos a ayudar.
   c. No se preocupe.
4. You are surrounded by family members all talking at once.
   a. No comprendo.
   b. Más despacio.
   c. Siéntese.

II. Dialogue

AUDIO CD

You will hear/read a series of dialogues in which you have arrived at a scene and have determined that no one will be able to translate for you.

You arrive at the scene of an auto accident.

EMT	**Señor, ¿habla inglés?**
Patient	**No, sólo hablo español.**
EMT	**Hablo un poco de español.**
Patient	**¡Ay! Estoy muy adolorido. Ayúdeme, por favor** *(Patient talks too fast.)*
EMT	**Por favor, no comprendo. Tengo unas preguntas.** *(Here the paramedic begins to ask his questions.)*

Translation

EMT	Sir, do you speak English?
Patient	No, I don't speak English.
EMT	Ok, I speak a little Spanish.
Patient	Oh, I'm in a lot of pain. Please help me.
EMT	Please, I don't understand. I have questions.

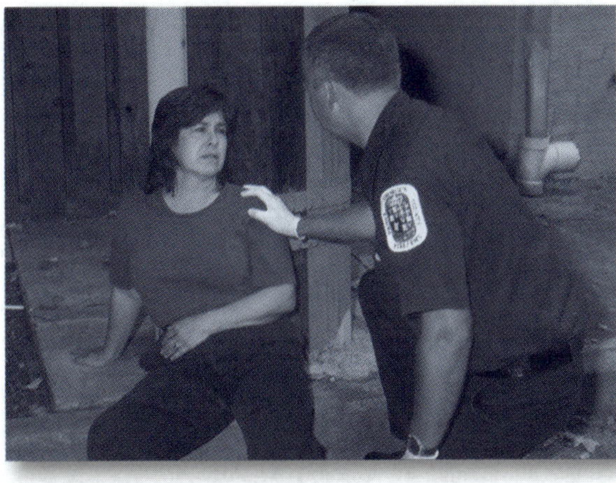

You arrive at the home of a family and the mother has burned herself badly. The children are frightened. No one speaks English.

EMT	Soy paramédico. Vamos a ayudar.
Child	¡Ay, ay Mami se quemó. ¿Se va a morir?
EMT	Cálmese, cálmese. Vamos a ayudar.
Mother	¡Ay! ¡Qué dolor! Déme algo para el dolor.
EMT	Silencio, por favor. Necesito examinarla.

Translation

EMT	I'm a paramedic. We're going to help.
Child	Oh, oh. Mom is burned. Is she going to die?
EMT	Calm down, calm down. We are going to help.
Mother	Oh! It hurts a lot! I need something for the pain.
EMT	Silence, please. I need to examine you.

You have arrived at the site of a fight. There are several men who may have been hurt.

EMT	Soy paramédico. ¿Quién necesita ayuda?
Patient 1	Yo. Estoy sangrando del brazo. Ese hombre me cortó.
EMT	¿Dónde está el cuchillo?
Patient 2	Allí. Yo también estoy herido.
EMT	Bien. Siéntese aquí y no se mueva. *(The men keep talking and yelling.)* Silencio, por favor. No comprendo. Tengo unas preguntas.

Translation

EMT	I'm a paramedic. Who needs help?
Patient 1	Me. My arm is bleeding. That man cut me.
EMT	Where is the knife?
Patient 2	There. I am also hurt.
EMT	Ok. Sit here and don't move. *(The men keep talking and yelling.)* Quiet, please. I don't understand. I have some questions.

You arrive at the home of a family with a sick child.

EMT	Soy paramédico. Vamos a ayudar.
Mother	Mi hijo ha estado vomitando.
EMT	No comprendo. ¿Es usted la mamá?
Mother	Sí, sí. Mi hijo está vomitando. *(Mother demonstrates vomiting.)*
EMT	Ah ¿vomita? ¿Mucho o poco?
Mother	Mucho. Tiene la gripe, el "flu."
EMT	Vamos a ayudar. No se preocupe.

Translation

EMT	I'm a paramedic. We're going to help.
Mother	My son has been vomiting.
EMT	I don't understand. Are you the mother?
Mother	Yes, yes. My son is vomiting. *(Mother demonstrates vomiting.)*
EMT	Ah, vomiting? A lot or a little?
Mother	A lot. He has the flu.
EMT	We're going to help. Don't worry.

AUDIO CD

III. Practice

Write and say in English the translations of the following Spanish phrases. Remember that you may do the exercise as often as it is necessary to become comfortable with it. Don't limit yourself to practicing it only once.

1. Silencio, por favor. ______________________
2. Tengo unas preguntas. ______________________
3. Más despacio. ______________________
4. Vamos a ayudar. ______________________
5. Cálmese. ______________________
6. Siéntese. ______________________
7. No se preocupe. ______________________
8. No comprendo. ______________________
9. Mucho o poco. ______________________
10. ¿Quién necesita ayuda? ______________________
11. Soy paramédico. ______________________

12. Hablo un poco de español. ____________________

13. ¿Es usted la mamá? ____________________

Now, you will be given just a phrase to translate to Spanish. These will later be combined to form whole questions and/or sentences. This is a good way to memorize, just a little bit at a time.

1. A little ____________
2. Of Spanish ____________
3. I speak ____________
4. Help ____________
5. Needs ____________
6. Who ____________
7. To help ____________
8. We're going ____________
9. A paramedic ____________
10. I am ____________
11. Please ____________
12. Sit down ____________

Take the vocabulary from the previous exercise and combine the words to form some of the phrases and questions. Repeat the answer several times.

1. I speak a little Spanish. ____________________
2. Who needs help? ____________________
3. We're going to help. ____________________
4. I'm a paramedic. ____________________
5. Sit down, please. ____________________

Now, we will do the same type of exercise but this time you will be providing the Spanish. This will be more difficult but don't give up and remember that you may divide the exercise into smaller portions. For example, you may want to work through the first six several times before going on to the rest. Also, whenever possible, be sure to write as well as to say the answers.

1. I don't understand. ____________________
2. I speak a little Spanish. ____________________
3. Calm down. ____________________
4. Slower, please. ____________________
5. Don't worry. ____________________

6. Who needs help? ______________________________

7. I'm a paramedic. ______________________________

8. We're going to help. ______________________________

9. Sit down, please. ______________________________

10. A lot or a little? ______________________________

11. I have questions. ______________________________

12. Quiet, please. ______________________________

What responses would you give to the following situations? There may be more than one possible answer.

1. You wish to reassure the patient that you are going to help him because you are a paramedic. ______________________________

2. You understand that the patient is in pain and you wish to know how severe it is. ______________________________

3. You want the patient to calm down and sit. ______________________________

4. You can't understand the patient but you need to ask some questions. ______________________________

IV. Vocabulary 2

The following are phrases and words that were presented in the earlier dialogues that you might hear at the scene. Listen and read these phrases so that you may become familiar with them. Memorization is not necessary but it is a good idea to have an idea of what the patients may be saying.

Ayuda	Help
Ayúdeme	Help me
Dolor	Pain
¡Qué dolor!	It hurts! (How it hurts!)
Está sangrando.	He/she is/ you are bleeding.
Está vomitando.	He/she is/ you are vomiting.
Me duele.	It hurts.
Sangre	Blood
Se quemó.	He/she burned him/herself.
Tiene (la gripe).	He/she has (the flu).
Yo también	I also (me, too)
Estoy herido(a).	I'm hurt.

Read the following phrases that patients and bystanders are saying and then translate to English.

1. ¡Ay! Tengo mucho dolor. ____________________
2. Me duele aquí. ____________________
3. ¡Ay, no! Está sangrando mucho. ____________________
4. ¡Qué dolor! Ayúdeme, ayúdeme. ____________________
5. Está vomitando. Tiene la gripe. ____________________

V. Review

Go back and listen again to the dialogues. How well are you able to understand what the people are saying? You should notice that you understand quite a bit now. Great job! Think of the phrases and questions that will be helpful to you from this chapter. Write them down on cards and begin keeping a file of them in order to review daily. You're now ready to move on to the next chapter.

VI. Cultural Capsule

Hispanics and Latinos in the United States

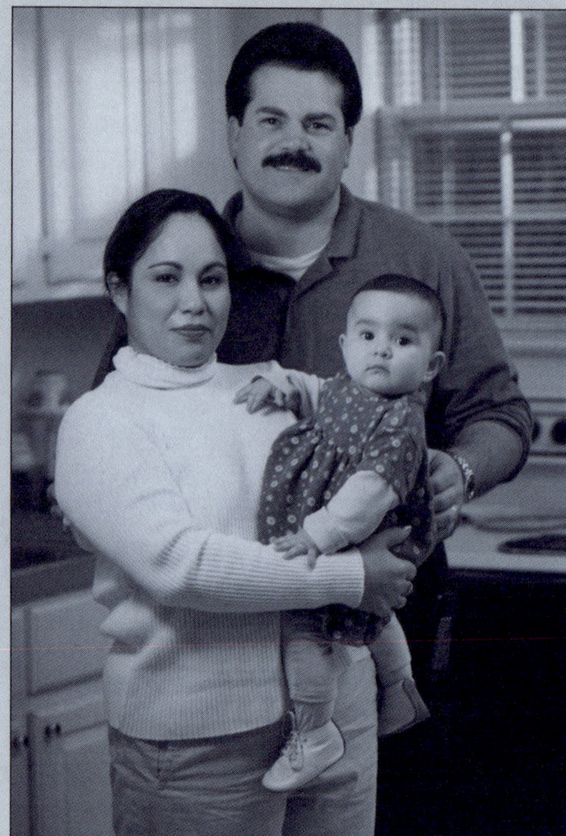

Today there are 25 to 30 million Hispanics and Latinos living in the United States, and Spanish is the second most spoken language. Many Hispanics and Latinos have become "Americanized" but others, especially the elderly or newly emigrated, still cling to their heritage and language. In many cities there are pockets of "Spanish only" sections where Hispanics are able to live without ever using English as they go about their daily affairs. While many immigrants are thankful for being in the United States, some find it difficult to embrace a new culture that is so very different from that of their native country.

The terms "Hispanic" and "Latino" encompass a large group of people who are from different countries, cultures, and backgrounds. Although there are similarities due to a common language and historical background, it is a mistake to try to fit all Hispanics and Latinos into one mold.

Reasons for immigrating to the United States vary from nationality to nationality. Cubans, living mainly in Miami and the northeast, have come to this country fleeing Castro's communism. Puerto Ricans, also settling mainly in the northeast, are citizens of the United States and may move freely between the island and the mainland. Many Puerto Ricans came to the mainland for economic reasons and have remained, raising their families here. Mexican-Americans are found throughout the United States, but are most prevalent in the Southwest. Some Mexican-American families have lived on homesteads since the early nineteenth century, while others have immigrated more recently. There are also other groups of Hispanic and Latino immigrants who come from the Caribbean, Central America, South America, or Spain.

While many Hispanics and Latinos immigrate to the United States for political or economic reasons, many others also come to study, to travel or simply to experience a different culture. Just as the United States is diverse as a whole, the Hispanic and Latino communities are diverse, complex, and dynamic.

Chapter 2

Accident at Home

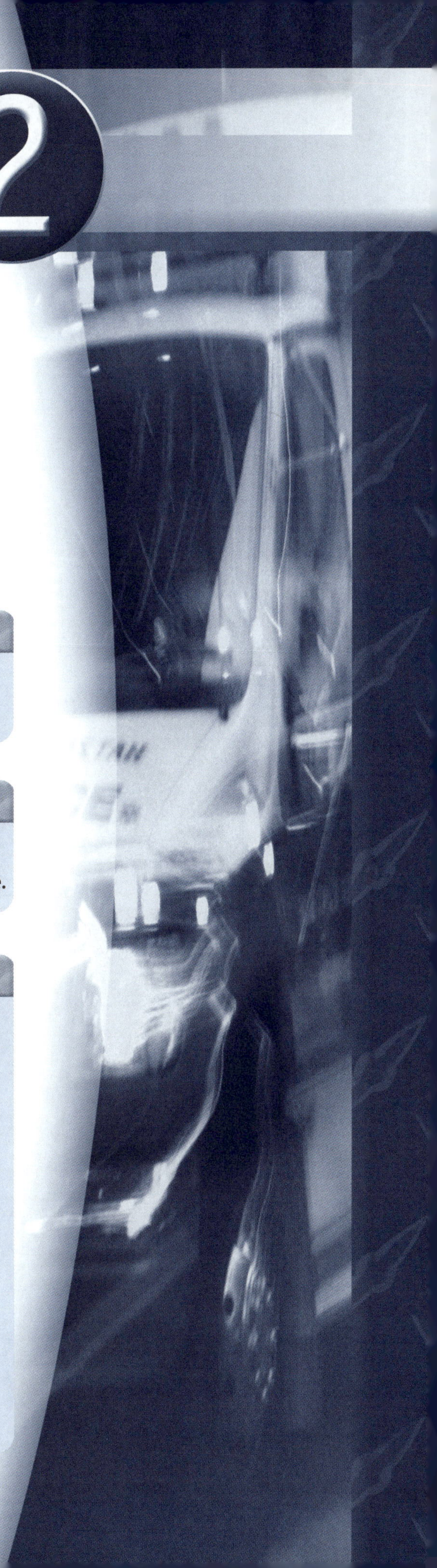

I. Vocabulary 1

AUDIO CD

Repeat the following words and phrases. Take your time and go over them several times before you move on to the next exercise. Remember to go over the first five a few times before moving on.

Commands

Señale dónde le duele.	Point to where it hurts.
Mire para arriba.	Look up.

Statements

Necesito tomarle el pulso.	I need to take your pulse.
Necesito tomarle la presión.	I need to take your blood pressure.

Questions

¿Dónde le duele?	Where does it hurt?
¿Es el dolor fuerte o débil?*	Is the pain strong or weak?
¿Se cayó?	Did you fall?
¿Cuándo ocurrió? ¿Hoy?	When did it happen? Today?
¿Cómo ocurrió?	How did it happen?
¿Fue un accidente?	Was it an accident?
¿Perdió el conocimiento?	Did you lose consciousness?
¿Ha comido hoy?	Have you eaten today?
¿Tiene náusea?	Are you nauseated?
¿Tiene adormecida alguna parte del cuerpo?	Do you have any numbness in any part of your body?
¿Tiene alergias a alguna medicina?	Do you have allergies to medicines?

* *Leve, débil, and suave can all be used to describe a weak or a slight pain.*

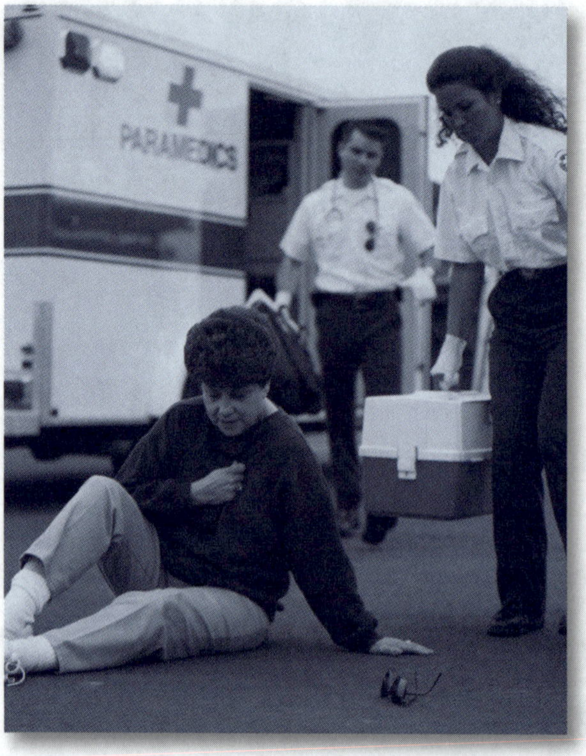

Review

Cálmese.	Calm down.
Vamos a ayudar.	We're going to help.

AUDIO CD

Repeat the following question words and their corresponding questions. Translate the questions to English and visualize an occasion where you would need to use them.

1. ¿Cómo?	How	¿Cómo ocurrió?	How did it happen?
2. ¿Cuándo?	When	¿Cuándo ocurrió?	When did it happen?
3. ¿Dónde?	Where	¿Dónde le duele?	Where does it hurt?
		¿Dónde tiene el dolor?	Where is the pain?

What questions would you ask to obtain the information below? Be sure to repeat the answers in Spanish.

1. How the person got hurt. ______________________

2. Where the person is hurt. ______________________

3. When the person got hurt. ______________________

Repeat the following commands. Translate the commands to English and visualize an occasion when you would need them.

1. Señale ____________ Señale dónde le duele. ____________
2. Cálmese ____________ Cálmese, por favor. ____________
3. Siéntese ____________ Siéntese aquí, por favor. ____________
4. Mire ____________ Mire para arriba. Míreme. ____________

Match the following English translations to the phrases presented in the previous exercise. Be sure to repeat the answer aloud in Spanish.

1. I need to take your pulse. ____________
2. Is the pain strong or weak? ____________
3. Did you eat today? ____________
4. Do you have allergies to medicines? ____________
5. Point to where it hurts. ____________
6. Do you feel any numbness? ____________
7. Are you nauseated? ____________

AUDIO CD

II. Dialogue

You arrive at a home where a woman is complaining of being in pain. She is clutching her head and is disoriented. You believe that she may have fallen from a ladder. An older woman keeps pointing and is speaking very rapidly.

EMT **Cálmese y siéntese, señora. Vamos a ayudar.**
Patient **Ayúdeme, por favor.**
EMT **Sí, señora. Vamos a ayudar. Señale dónde le duele.**
Patient **Aquí en la cabeza. Aquí en el estómago y aquí en la espalda.** *(She points.)*
EMT **¿Cómo es el dolor? ¿Fuerte o leve?**
Patient **Fuerte. Muy fuerte.**
EMT **¿Se cayó?**
Patient **Sí.**
EMT **¿Cuándo ocurrió? ¿Hoy?**
Patient **Sí, sí. Esta mañana.**
EMT **¿Cómo ocurrió? ¿Fue un accidente?**
Patient **Sí, me caí de la escalera.**

(Continued on next page)

EMT	¿Perdió el conocimiento?
Patient	Sí, por un momento.
EMT	¿Tiene náusea?
Patient	Sí.
EMT	¿Tiene adormecidas las manos y los pies?
Patient	No.
EMT	¿Tiene alergias a alguna medicina?
Patient	No.
EMT	¿Ha comido hoy?
Patient	Sí.
EMT	Necesito tomarle el pulso y la presión.
Patient	Bien. ¿Me va a dar algo para el dolor?
EMT	Silencio, por favor. *(EMT takes pulse and blood pressure.)* Mire para arriba. *(EMT checks her eyes.)* Vamos al hospital. ¿Bien?

Translation

EMT	Calm down and sit, ma'am. We're going to help.
Patient	Help me, please.
EMT	Yes, ma'am, we're going to help. Point to where it hurts.
Patient	Here, on my head. Here on my stomach and here on my back.
EMT	How is the pain? Strong or weak?
Patient	Strong, very strong.
EMT	Did you fall?
Patient	Yes.
EMT	When did it happen? Today?
Patient	Yes, yes. This morning.
EMT	How did it happen? An accident?
Patient	Yes, I fell from the ladder.
EMT	Did you lose consciousness?
Patient	Yes, for a moment.
EMT	Do you feel nauseated?
Patient	Yes.
EMT	Do you have numbness in your hands and feet?
Patient	No.
EMT	Do you have allergies to medicines?
Patient	No.
EMT	Did you eat today?
Patient	Yes.
EMT	I need to take your pulse and blood pressure.
Patient	Ok. Are you going to give me something for the pain?
EMT	Please, quiet. Look up. We're going to the hospital. Ok?

III. Practice

Translate the following words from Spanish to English. Be sure to write the words as well as say them.

1. Dolor ______________
2. Paramédico ______________
3. Pulso ______________
4. Presión ______________
5. Fuerte ______________
6. Débil ______________
7. Hospital ______________
8. Alergias ______________
9. Hoy ______________
10. Aquí ______________
11. Medicina ______________
12. Conocimiento ______________
13. Náusea ______________
14. Adormecido(a) ______________
15. Se cayó ______________
16. Cuerpo ______________

Now, translate the following words from English to Spanish. Again, write and repeat your responses.

1. Strong ______________
2. Today ______________
3. Pain ______________
4. Paramedic ______________
5. Pulse ______________
6. Here ______________
7. Weak ______________
8. Consciousness ______________
9. Allergies ______________
10. Hospital ______________
11. Blood pressure ______________
12. Medicine ______________
13. Fell ______________
14. Numbness ______________
15. Nauseated ______________

Using the words above, fill in the blanks and say the completed sentence aloud. Repeat the correct answer.

1. Necesito tomarle el ______________ y la ______________.
2. ¿Tiene ______________ a alguna medicina?
3. El ______________ es fuerte, no ______________.
4. No se preocupe. Vamos al ______________.
5. ¿Perdió el ______________ hoy?

Translate the following sentences to English. Remember to say them aloud as well.

1. ¿Cuándo ocurrió? ______
2. ¿Hoy? ______
3. ¿Dónde le duele? ______
4. ¿Aquí? ______
5. ¿Cómo es el dolor? ______
6. ¿Fuerte o débil? ______
7. ¿Perdió el conocimiento? ______
8. ¿Ha comido hoy? ______
9. Vamos al hospital. ______
10. Vamos a ayudar. ______
11. Necesito tomarle el pulso. ______
12. Necesito tomarle la presión. ______
13. ¿Tiene alergias? ______
14. ¿Tiene medicinas? ______
15. Mire para arriba. ______
16. ¿Tiene adormecida alguna parte del cuerpo? ______
17. ¿Tiene náusea? ______

Using the above vocabulary, how would you respond to the following situations?

1. Tell the patient that you need to take his blood pressure and pulse. ______
2. Ask the patient if he has eaten today. ______
3. Ask the patient where it hurts. ______

4. Ask the patient if the pain is strong or weak. ____________________

5. Ask the patient if he lost consciousness. ____________________

6. Ask the patient when it happened. Today? ____________________

7. Ask the patient if he has any allergies or medicines. ____________________

8. Tell the patient you are going to help. ____________________

9. Tell the patient you are going to the hospital. ____________________

10. Tell the patient to calm down. ____________________

11. Tell the patient not to worry. ____________________

12. Tell the bystanders to be quiet. ____________________

13. Ask the patient to point to where it hurts. ____________________

14. Ask the patient if he has any numbness. ____________________

15. Ask the patient if he is nauseated. ____________________

Let's take a look at some of the "key" verbs that you have been using. Repeat and translate the following list. After you have gone through this exercise, jot down some of the questions and phrases that you have been using with these verbs.

1. Vamos a We're going to ____________________
2. Necesito I need (to) ____________________

3. Tiene Do you have (Does he/she have)? ______

4. Duele Hurt ______

5. Perdió Did you lose? ______

IV. Vocabulary 2: What Patients and Bystanders Might Say

Listen and repeat the following vocabulary. Remember that the main purpose is for you to recognize the words and phrases when you hear them spoken.

Aquí	Here	Ocurrió	It happened
No es	Is not	Me caí.	I fell.
En	In, on	La escalera	The ladder
Estómago	Stomach	Perdí el conocimiento.	I lost consciousness.
Dolor	Pain	Me duele el estómago.	My stomach hurts.
Cabeza	Head	Me duele la cabeza.	My head hurts.
Espalda	Back	Me duela la espalda.	My back hurts.
Esta mañana	This morning		

Provide a possible question or phrase you might have asked or said that caused the following responses.

1. You: ______

   Patient: Aquí. Me duele la espalda. *(Patient points.)*

2. You: ______

   Patient: El dolor no es muy fuerte. Es leve.

3. You: ______

   Patient: Ocurrió esta mañana.

4. You: ______

   Patient: Sí, tengo alergia a la penicilina.

5. You: ______

   Patient: No, no perdí el conocimiento.

V. Review

At this point you may wish to review by listening again to the dialogue. This will keep training your ear to the Spanish sounds and pronunciation. Remember to jot down the questions and phrases that you find particularly useful on cards and keep practicing. You're doing great!

VI. Cultural Capsule

Understanding Differences

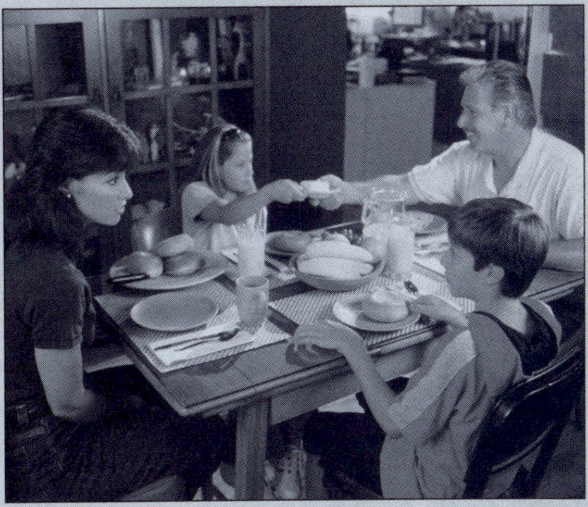

In treating patients in the field, it is necessary to be aware of preconceived ideas about Hispanics and Latinos. This is especially true if stereotyping interferes in the medical treatment of patients. Stereotyping arises from a lack of understanding of a different culture. It is true that differences do exist, but so do similarities. By being aware of both the differences and similarities of a culture, understanding follows.

Hispanics and Latinos include people of Caucasian, African, Asian, Native American, and biracial descent. Some speak only Spanish, others only English, and many are bilingual. Hispanics and Latinos face prejudice and discrimination on many levels: race, ethnicity, socioeconomic class, legal status, and education.

When Hispanics and Latinos are faced with a medical emergency, should their first contact be one tainted by prejudice or one that instills a sense of trust? Hispanics have a saying, "*el mundo es un pañuelo,*" which literally means, "the world is a handkerchief." In English there is a similar saying, "It's a small world." Different words from different cultures, but with the same meaning, can be found in both sayings.

Chapter 3

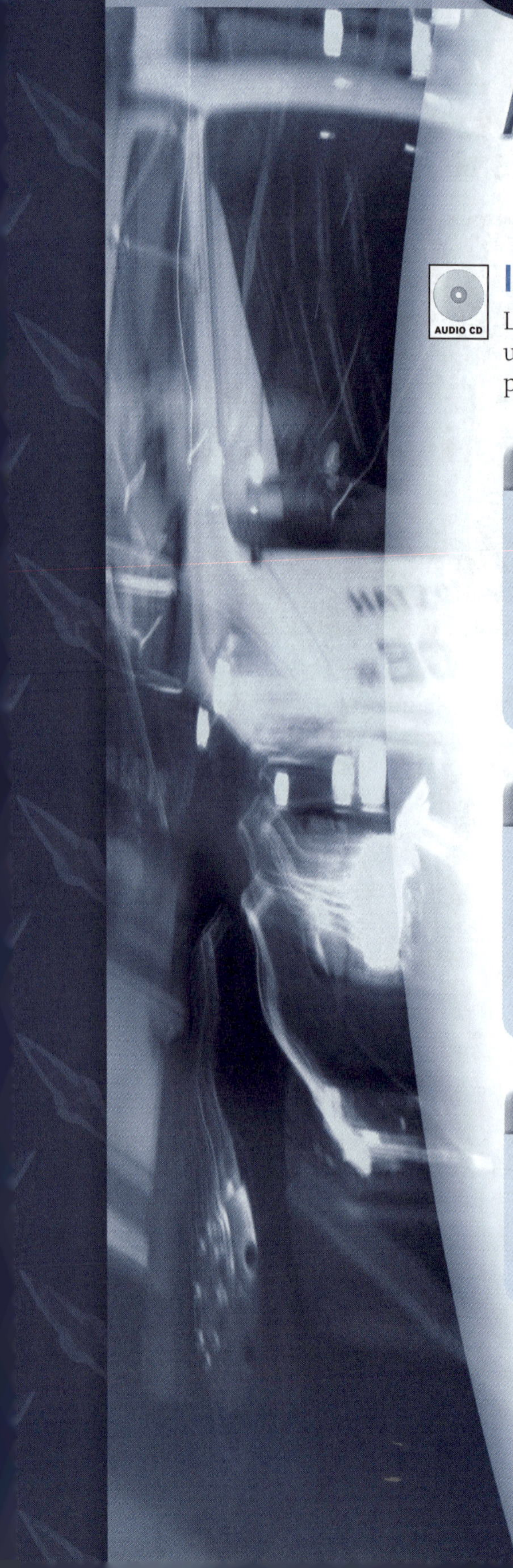

Assault

I. Vocabulary 1

AUDIO CD

Listen and repeat the following vocabulary. Always visualize yourself using the phrases on the scene. Remember to practice only a few of the phrases at a time before you move on.

Commands

Siéntese, por favor.	Sit down, please.
Señale dónde está herido.	Point to where you are wounded.
Muévase, por favor.	Move, please.
Acuéstese en la camilla.	Lay down on the stretcher.
Cálmese.	Calm down.
No se preocupe.	Don't worry.

Statements

Necesito tomarle el pulso.	I need to take your pulse.
Necesito tomarle la presión.	I need to take your blood pressure.
Vamos al hospital.	We're going to the hospital.
No hablo español.	I don't speak Spanish.
Gracias.	Thank you.

Questions

¿Cuándo ocurrió?	When did it happen?
¿Minutos? ¿Horas?	Minutes? Hours?
¿Dónde está el cuchillo? ¿la pistola?	Where is the knife? the gun?

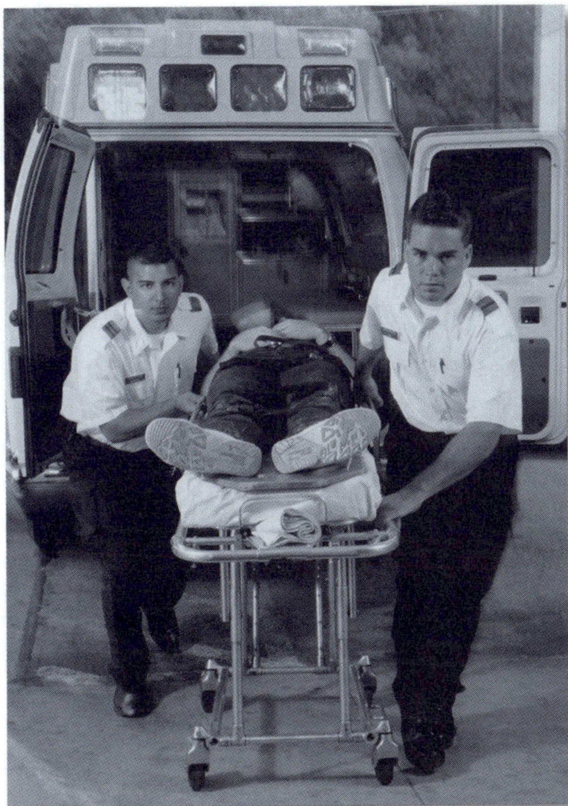

Let's review a few of the commands presented above. What do the following words mean in English?

1. Cálmese ____________________
2. Señale ____________________
3. Siéntese ____________________
4. Muévase ____________________
5. No se preocupe ____________________
6. Acuéstese ____________________

What would you say in the following situations? More than one answer is possible. Be sure to repeat the answers. You want to do this exercise a couple of times before moving on.

1. You need to tell someone to move. ____________________
2. You need to tell the patient to lay down on the stretcher. ____________________
3. You need to know where someone is wounded. ____________________
4. You want to know when something happened. Hours, minutes? ____________________
5. You're going to take the patient's pulse and blood pressure. ____________________

II. Dialogue

You arrive at a scene where two men have been in a fight. One of the men is yelling and will not sit down.

EMT Por favor, silencio. Siéntese.

Patient ¡Ay! ¡Qué dolor!

EMT Por favor. Siéntese. Vamos a ayudar.

Patient *(Patient sits down and quiets down.)*

EMT ¿Dónde está el cuchillo?

Patient Aquí. *(Hands over the knife.)*

EMT Gracias. Señale dónde está herido.

Patient Me cortó aquí en el brazo y aquí en la pierna.

EMT Bien. Necesito tomarle el pulso y la presión. *(Patient is quiet.)* Por favor, acuéstese en la camilla. Vamos al hospital.

Patient ¡Ay! ¿Estoy bien? ¿Qué pasa?

EMT Cálmese. No se preocupe. Vamos al hospital.

Translation

EMT Please, be quiet. Sit down.

Patient Oh! What terrible pain!

EMT Please sit down. We're going to help.

Patient *(Patient sits down and quiets down.)*

EMT Where is the knife?

Patient Here. *(Hands over the knife.)*

EMT Thank you. Point to where you are wounded.

Patient He cut me here on my arm and here on my leg.

EMT Ok. I need to take your pulse and your blood pressure. *(Patient is quiet.)* Please lay down on the stretcher. We're going to the hospital.

Patient Oh! Am I ok? What's going on?

EMT Calm down. Don't worry. We're going to the hospital.

A man has been shot. He is unconscious. No one speaks English and the family is all around talking and crying. Several people are blocking the way to the patient.

EMT Por favor, silencio. Vamos a ayudar. *(The family quiets down but is still hovering over the man.)*

EMT Por favor, ¿dónde está la pistola? *(Someone points to where the gun is and says, "Allí.")*

EMT Por favor, muévase. Vamos a ayudar. *(EMTs check the patient and put him on a backboard.)*

EMT ¿Cuándo ocurrió? ¿Hace cuántas horas o minutos? *(EMT indicates with his or her fingers the number of hours or minutes.)*

EMT Gracias, vamos al hospital.

(Continued on next page)

Translation

EMT	Please, silence. We're going to help.
EMT	Please, where is the gun?
EMT	Please, move. We're going to help.
EMT	When did it happen? Hours? Minutes?
EMT	Thank you, we're going to the hospital.

AUDIO CD

III. Practice

Translate the following words and phrases found in Vocabulary 1 from English to Spanish. Remember to repeat the correct answer.

1. Hospital ______
2. Sit down. ______
3. Move ______
4. Thank you ______
5. Stretcher ______
6. Wounded ______
7. Hours ______
8. Minutes ______
9. I need ______
10. Silence ______
11. Knife ______
12. Gun ______

AUDIO CD

Translate the following sentences and questions from English to Spanish. Remember to do only two or three at a time, repeat several times and then go on to the next set of two or three.

1. Point to where you are wounded. ______
2. Sit down, please. ______
3. Calm down. ______
4. I need to take your pulse and blood pressure. ______
5. Lay down on the stretcher, please. ______
6. When did it occur? ______
7. Move, please. ______
8. Don't worry. ______
9. Where is the knife? ______
10. We're going to the hospital. ______

What would you say in the following situations? More than one answer is possible. Be sure to repeat the answer and remember that there are several possibilities.

1. You arrive at a scene where everyone is talking, very upset, and hovering over the patient. ____________________
2. You need to determine where the patient is hurt or wounded. ____________________
3. You need for the patient to lay down on the stretcher. ____________________
4. You want to know when something happened. ____________________
5. You want to tell the patient you're going to the hospital. ____________________
6. You want to reassure the patient. ____________________

AUDIO CD

Translate the following commands from English to Spanish. Be sure to do the exercise several times until you have mastered the material.

1. Calm down. ____________
2. Quiet. ____________
3. Sit down. ____________
4. Lay down. ____________
5. Move. ____________
6. Point. ____________

AUDIO CD

IV. Vocabulary 2

Repeat the following vocabulary. Become familiar with the sound of the words and phrases. You may not have to use them yourself but you may hear the patients use them.

¿Estoy bien?	Am I ok?
¿Qué pasa?	What's happening?
Me cortó.	He/she cut me.
El brazo	The arm
La pierna	The leg
¡Qué dolor! ¡Me duele mucho!	How painful! (It really hurts!)

What would you have said to elicit the following responses from patients? Remember to repeat the correct answer.

1. You: ____________________

   Patient: Me cortó aquí en la pierna y aquí en el brazo.

2. You: ____________________

   Patient: *(Lies down on the stretcher.)*

3. You: ____________________

   Patient: *(Bystander moves away from patient.)*

V. Review

In this section, it is all up to you and your experience. Pick out at least 10 statements and/or questions from the first three chapters that you think will be helpful to you personally when you are at a scene of an assault. Write them down on the cards if you haven't already done this. Now, think of what the patients might say and do when you say these things to them. Are there any additional questions or statements that you might need? Are there some that are not included? Can you construct them yourself with the vocabulary given so far or do you need to refer to Appendix A? Don't worry if the phrases don't come immediately to mind. A foreign language is a skill and it takes practice. So, just review what you have learned so far and move on to the next chapter.

VI. Cultural Capsule

Different Cultures, Different Emotional Responses

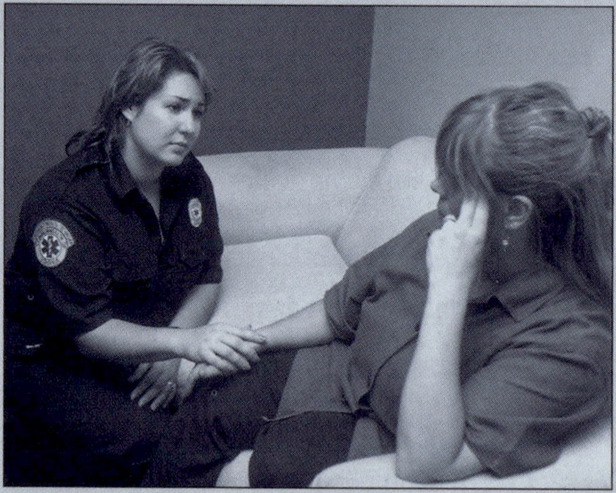

There are a few differences that may cause a North American to misinterpret the situation or become frustrated or annoyed with a Hispanic's or Latino's response to an emergency. Some have to do with the basic control of a scene. A medic wishes to bring some order and calm into a chaotic situation and may sometimes find the emotions displayed by some Hispanic patients and their family members somewhat overwhelming. Although the scene may benefit from everyone being calm, it may be necessary to reassure the family members in a way that engenders in them a sense of trust or confidence in the medic.

This sense of confidence and trust, known in Spanish as "confianza" is a very important part in acceptance of a caregiver. In order to build "confianza" in Hispanic patients or their families, it is essential that a person be polite and reassuring.

Unfortunately, in some cases, the medic has already engendered a certain distrust or fear in the patient simply by wearing a uniform. The uniforms may have negative connotations for those who left countries where either government troops or guerrilla fighters were constantly threatening the population. Added to this are the illegal aliens whose fear of the Border Patrol or Immigration is paramount. Such a simple thing as introducing yourself and asking for someone's name can build a bridge between the medic and the patient. Do not be surprised, however, if trust does not come right away.

Another point of frustration at times is the issue of eye contact. In some Latino cultures it is impolite to look someone in the eye, especially if the person is viewed as someone in power. As the medic, you are in charge and will be treated as such. Looking away is not a sign of being dishonest or of being inattentive, but rather it is a sign of respect. Of course, not all Latino cultures view eye contact differently from North Americans. As the medic works in his or her community, it will become evident whether eye contact is an issue or not.

A frustrating situation for medics who are natives of the United States is the overcrowding of a scene. Not only does the medic need space in which to work, but he or she also needs a certain amount of personal space so as to feel comfortable. The amount of personal space people need is governed by what their culture deems as appropriate. Many Hispanic and Latino immigrants who have not yet assimilated fully into the North American culture require less personal space than someone raised in the United States or Canada. The people around the scene, therefore, may not realize that they are crowding the medic and making him or her uncomfortable. If the medic needs the space, he or she should simply ask politely, *"Por favor, necesito más espacio para trabajar,"* (Please, I need more space in which to work).

Hispanics and Latinos recognize that there are differences in their culture that can be confusing to North Americans. With some understanding on both parts, a chaotic and frightening situation can be brought under control for the benefit of the patient.

Chapter 4

An Auto Accident

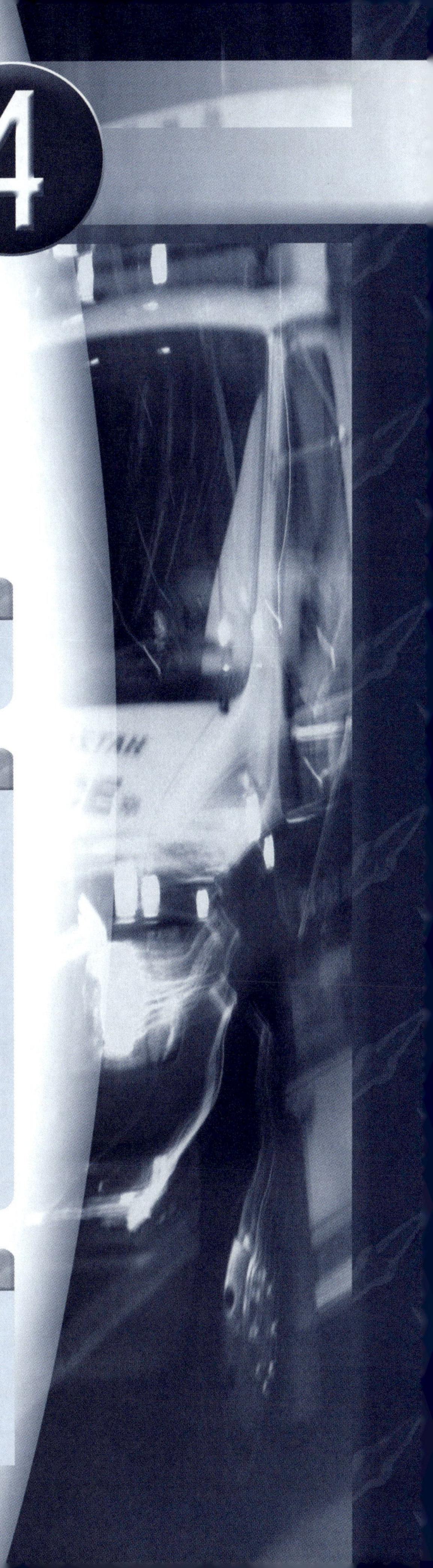

I. Vocabulary 1

AUDIO CD

Repeat the following phrases. Remember to work with a few at a time before moving on to the next set.

Commands	
Señale dónde le duele.	Point to where it hurts.
Escriba el nombre.	Write down the name.

Statements	
No comprendo.	I don't understand.
Necesito tomarle ______.	I need to take ______.
Necesito ponerle ______.	I need to put on ______.
Tengo unas preguntas.	I have questions.
Un collar ortopédico	A neck brace
Una tablilla	A splint
Vamos a ayudar.	We're going to help.
Vamos a la camilla.	Let's go to the stretcher.
Necesito ponerle ______.	I need to put on ______.
Un collar ortopédico	A neck brace
Una tablilla	A splint
Vamos a la camilla.	Let's go to the stretcher.
Es necesario.	It is necessary.

Questions	
¿Es el dolor fuerte o leve (suave, débil)?	Is the pain strong or weak?
¿Es el dolor agudo?	Is the pain sharp?
¿Se extiende el dolor?	Does the pain extend out?

(Continued on next page)

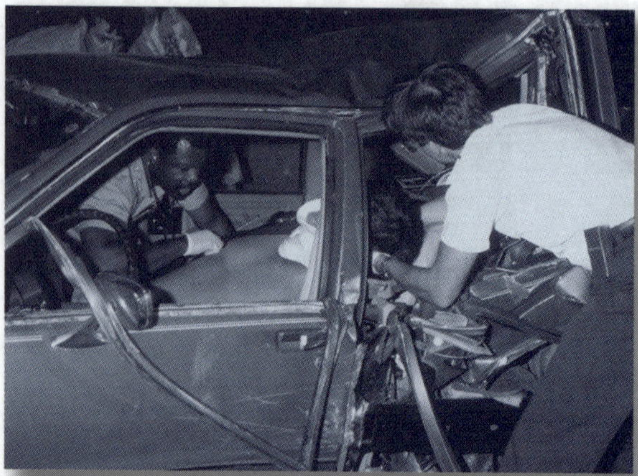

¿Quién necesita ayuda?	Who needs help?
¿Tiene alergias a alguna medicina?	Do you have allergies to medicines?
¿Toma medicinas? ¿Qué?	Do you take medicines? What?
¿Qué hospital prefiere?	What hospital do you prefer?

Let's review a few of the nouns in this section. Write the English translation.

1. Ayuda ____________
2. Dolor ____________
3. Alergias ____________
4. Medicinas ____________
5. Collar ortopédico ____________
6. Tablilla ____________

Now we will translate from English to Spanish.

1. Allergies ____________
2. Medicines ____________
3. Help ____________
4. Neck brace ____________
5. Splint ____________
6. Pain ____________

Go through these situations several times until you are able to give a response quickly.

1. You arrive on the scene and want to know who needs help. ____________
____
2. Tell the patient to point to where it hurts. ____________
____

3. You want to assess the severity of the pain. ______________________________

____

4. You don't understand. ____________________

____

5. You want information on allergies and medicines. ______________________

____

6. You need to put on a neck brace and a splint. ________________________

____

II. Dialogue

You have arrived at a scene of an auto accident and have determined that no one can translate for you.

EMT Vamos a ayudar. Hablo un poco de español.

Patient Ay, ay, ay. Por favor, ayúdeme.

EMT Sí, señora. ¿Quién necesita ayuda?

Patient Yo, señor. Me duele el cuello y estoy sangrando de la frente.

EMT Por favor, no comprendo. Señale dónde le duele.

Patient *(Pointing)* Aquí, señor. El cuello, la cabeza y el brazo. ¡Ay, ay, ay!

EMT Silencio, señora, por favor. *(The patient quiets down.)* Necesito tomarle la presión y el pulso.

Patient ¿Me voy a morir?

EMT Cálmese, señora. Silencio, por favor. *(EMT takes blood pressure and pulse.)* Tengo unas preguntas, señora.

Patient Sí, señor, ¿qué?

EMT ¿Es agudo el dolor? ¿Sí o no?

Patient No.

EMT ¿Se extiende?

Patient Sí.

EMT Señale por dónde.

Patient De aquí a aquí. *(Points around the neck area.)*

EMT ¿Es fuerte o leve el dolor?

Patient Fuerte.

EMT ¿Tiene alergias a alguna medicina?

Patient Sí.

EMT ¿Qué?

Patient Penicilina.

EMT Bien, ¿Está tomando alguna medicina ahora?

Patient Sí, para el corazón.

(Continued on next page)

EMT	Necesito la medicina, por favor.
Patient	No, no la tengo.
EMT	Escriba el nombre de la medicina. *(Patient writes down the name of the medicine.)* ¿Ha comido hoy?
Patient	Sí.
EMT	¿Qué hospital prefiere?
Patient	No me importa. El más cercano.
EMT	Necesito ponerle un collar ortopédico y una tablilla.
Patient	Ay, ¿me va a doler?
EMT	Cálmese, cálmese.
Patient	¡Ay! ¡Me duele!
EMT	Lo siento. Es necesario.
Patient	Está bien.
EMT	Vamos a ponerle en la camilla. Vamos al hospital.

Translation

EMT	We're going to help. I speak a little Spanish.
Patient	Oh, oh, oh. Please help me.
EMT	Yes, ma'am. Who needs help?
Patient	I do, sir. My neck hurts and I am bleeding from my forehead.
EMT	Please. I don't understand. Point to where it hurts.
Patient	*(Pointing.)* Here, sir. My neck, head, and arm. Oh, oh, oh!
EMT	Please, be silent, ma'am. *(The patient quiets down.)* I need to take your blood pressure and your pulse.
Patient	Am I going to die?
EMT	Calm down, ma'am. Please be silent. *(EMT takes blood pressure and pulse.)* I have some questions, ma'am.
Patient	Yes, sir. What?
EMT	Is the pain sharp? Yes or no?
Patient	No.
EMT	Does it radiate?
Patient	Yes.
EMT	Point to where.
Patient	Yes, from here to here. *(Points around the neck area.)*
EMT	Is the pain strong or weak?
Patient	Strong.
EMT	Do you have allergies to medicines?
Patient	Yes.
EMT	What?
Patient	Penicillin.
EMT	Are you taking any medicines now?
Patient	Yes, for my heart.
EMT	I need the medicine, please.
Patient	I don't have it.

(Continued on next page)

EMT	Write down the name of the medicine. *(Patient writes down the name of the medicine.)* Did you eat today?
Patient	Yes.
EMT	What hospital would you prefer?
Patient	It doesn't matter. The nearest one.
EMT	I need to put a neck brace and a splint on you.
Patient	Is it going to hurt? Oh!
EMT	Calm down, calm down.
Patient	Oh, it hurts!
EMT	I'm sorry. It's necessary.
Patient	Ok, ok.
EMT	We're going to put you on the stretcher. We're going to the hospital.

III. Practice

AUDIO CD

Translate the following words from Spanish to English. Be sure to say the word in Spanish as you practice it. Do this lesson a couple of times before moving on.

1. Preguntas ____________
2. Necesito ____________
3. Medicinas ____________
4. Prefiere ____________
5. Señale ____________
6. Ayuda ____________
7. Alergias ____________
8. Hospital ____________
9. Dolor ____________
10. Silencio ____________
11. Collar ortopédico ____________
12. Fuerte ____________
13. Débil ____________
14. Camilla ____________
15. Paramédico ____________

AUDIO CD

Translate the following phrases from English to Spanish. Remember these are found in Vocabulary 1. Practice a few phrases at a time until you are very comfortable.

1. I don't understand. ____________
2. Point to where it hurts. ____________
3. Is the pain sharp? ____________
4. Is the pain strong or weak? ____________

5. I have to put a neck brace on you. ____________________
6. We're going to put you on the stretcher. ____________________
7. Do you take any medicines? ____________________
8. What hospital do you prefer? ____________________
9. Who needs help? ____________________
10. Do you have any allergies to medicines? ____________________

Translate the following question words into English. Then, in the spaces provided, write a question using the word in Spanish (check Appendix A).

1. ¿Qué? ____________________
____
2. ¿Quién? ____________________
____

In the following exercise, the patient's response is given and you are to provide the question or phrase given by the medic. You may wish to repeat the answer several times.

1. You: ____________________
Patient: El dolor es muy fuerte.
2. You: ____________________
Patient: Sí, tengo alergia a la penicilina.
3. You: ____________________
Patient: Me duele aquí en el cuello y aquí en la cabeza.
4. You: ____________________
Patient: Sí, tomo "digital" para el corazón.
5. You: ____________________
Patient: Aquí, por favor, yo necesito ayuda.
6. You: ____________________
Patient: Prefiero ir al hospital más cercano.

Provide the response that you would give to the following situations. Remember to repeat the correct answers.

1. A patient is hysterical and talking too fast. ____________________
____

2. You're not sure who needs help. ______________________________

____

3. You need to find out where the patient is hurt. ______________________________

____

4. You need to find out what the pain is like. ______________________________

____

5. You need to find out what medicines the patient is taking. ______________________________

____

6. You ask the patient if she has a hospital preference. ______________________________

____

7. You tell the patient that what you're doing is necessary. ______________________________

____

8. You tell the patient that you're going to put a splint on him. ______________________________

____

9. You need to find out if the patient has eaten today. ______________________________

____

AUDIO CD

IV. Vocabulary 2

Below is a vocabulary list of the remarks made by the patient in the previous dialogue. Be sure to listen and become familiar with the words and phrases.

Ayúdeme.	Help me.
Estoy sangrando.	I'm bleeding.
Me duele el cuello.	My neck hurts.
Me duele la cabeza.	My head hurts.
¿Me voy a morir?	Am I going to die?
No importa.	It's not important/It doesn't matter.
Para el corazón	For the heart
Penicilina	Penicillin
Tomo una medicina (digital).	I take medicine (digitalis).

Provide the question or phrase that elicits the following responses from the patients or bystanders.

1. You: ______________________________

   Patient: Tomo una medicina para el corazón. La digital.

2. You: ______________________________

   Patient: Me duele el cuello y la cabeza.

3. You: ______________________________

   Patient: Sí, la penicilina.

V. Review

It's time to go back and listen again to the dialogue and keep your ear tuned to the sounds of Spanish. Also remember to keep adding to your card file. Daily exposure is very important. A good way to train your ear and treat yourself at the same time is to listen to some upbeat Spanish music. You may not understand the words but your brain is processing the sounds. Just enjoy and have fun with it!

VI. Cultural Capsule

Family

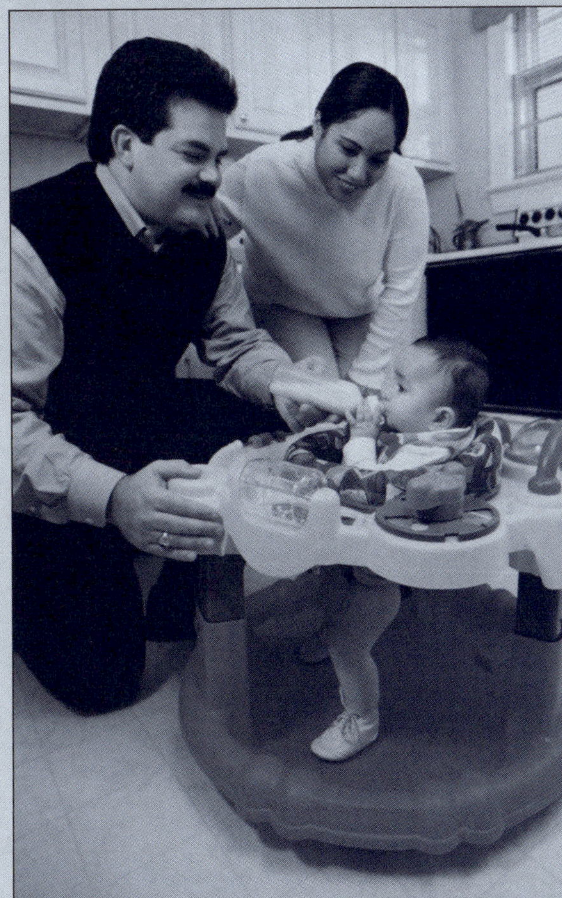

The importance of "la familia" to a Hispanic or Latino should never be underestimated. It is the core from which Hispanics get their strength. It is important to realize that the Latino family consists not only of the nuclear unit but also of an extended number of relatives, including grandparents, aunts, uncles, cousins and godparents. At times, even neighbors become assimilated into the family. It is possible for several members of the family to live together or at least very near each other.

The concept of "la familia" is important to the medic treating patients in the field because of the influence that the family will have on both the patient and on the situation. Quite often, it is thought that the patient, because he or she is hurt or ill, cannot make decisions regarding his or her care. The family will then take over. Often, the mother or grandmother will decide, since they are the ones in charge of nursing family members using home remedies. It is helpful to find out if the patient was given a "cocimiento," usually an herbal tea, or some other homemade remedy.

In controlling the scene, the medic will benefit from being aware that if one family member is hurt, everyone will wish to participate in the patient's recovery. The scene may feel overrun with family members and neighbors. They are not there as curious bystanders but as support for the patient. It is important for them to be there since the patient relies on their strength and counsel. Many will wish to travel to the hospital with the patient in the ambulance or will try to follow in a car. In some Latin American countries, the hospitals rely on the patients bringing their own linens. The medic may be faced, therefore, with well-meaning relatives insisting on bringing blankets and sheets for the patient.

Remember that the family is a great source of support for the patient and may also help the medic in trying to treat the patient. They will be eager to help in any way possible.

Chapter 5

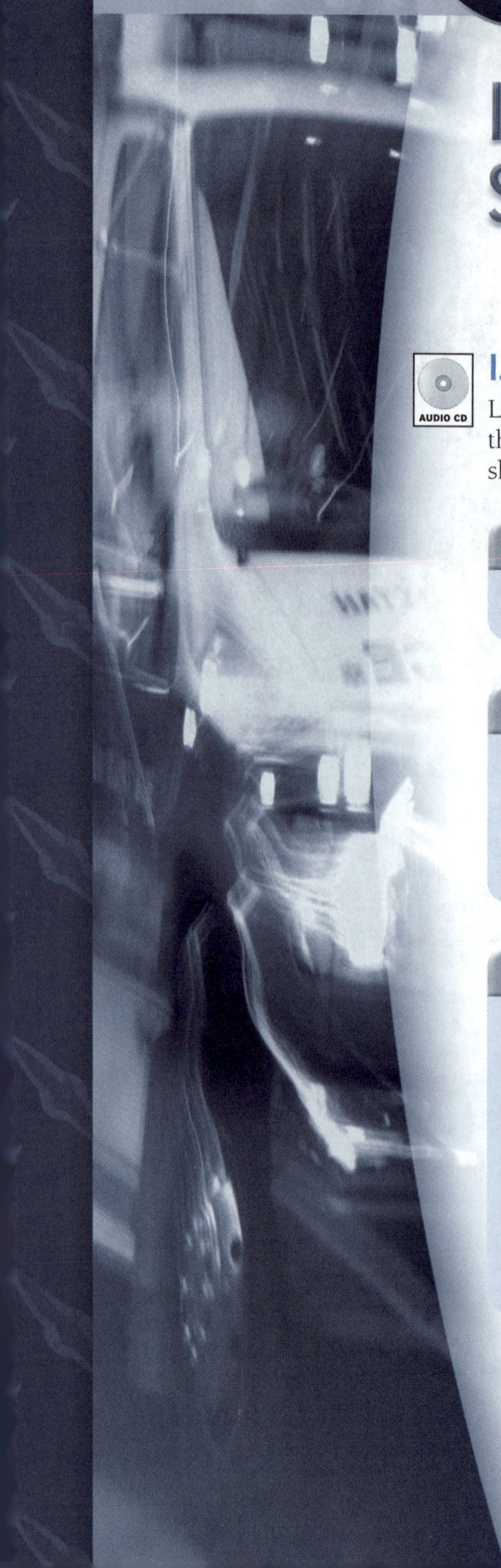

Illness 1: Stomach Ailments

I. Vocabulary 1

Listen and repeat the following phrases and questions. Remember to do this several times and to divide up the list. You're almost at the end and should be an old hand at this by now.

Commands	
No se preocupe.	Don't worry.

Statements	
Necesita líquidos.	You need liquids (he/she needs liquids).
Vamos a ponerle un suero.	We are going to start (put in) an IV.
No comprendo.	I don't understand.

Questions	
¿Qué le pasa?	What's the problem?
¿Le duele el estómago aquí?	Does your stomach hurt here?
¿Perdió el conocimiento?	Did you lose consciousness?
¿Tiene diarrea?	Do you have diarrhea?
¿Tiene vómitos?	Are you vomiting?
¿Tiene fiebre?	Do you have a fever?
¿Tiene una enfermedad crónica?	Do you have a chronic illness?
¿Qué hospital prefiere?	What hospital do you prefer?

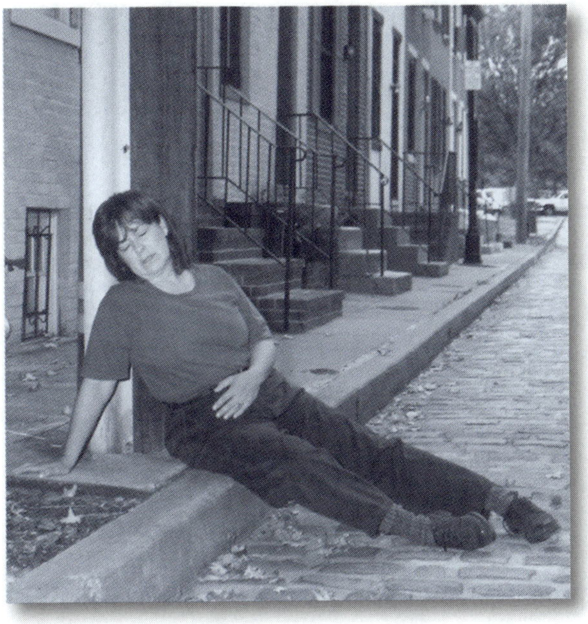

Give the English for the following words.

1. Conocimiento ____________
2. Líquidos ____________
3. Enfermedad ____________
4. Estómago ____________
5. Vómitos ____________
6. Suero ____________
7. Diarrea ____________
8. Crónica ____________
9. Fiebre ____________

Read the following situations and determine which of the above phrases or questions could be used in responding.

1. You want to know if the patient's stomach hurts. ____________
2. You want to know if the patient fainted (lost consciousness) earlier. ____________
3. You want to know if the patient is vomiting or has diarrhea. ____________
4. You tell the patient you are going to start an IV and he should not worry. ____________

AUDIO CD

II. Dialogue

Listen to the following dialogue until you are able to understand it without reading it at the same time. It will take several sessions so don't give up too soon.

You arrive at a home where you find a woman lying on the floor, looking very pale.

EMT	**Vamos a ayudar. ¿Qué le pasa?**
Patient	*(On floor and very pale.)* **Me desmayé. Vomité y tengo dolor de estómago.**
EMT	**No comprendo. ¿Le duele el estómago?**
Patient	**Sí, tengo mucho dolor. ¡Ay!**
EMT	**¿Le duele aquí?**
Patient	**Sí, sí. ¡Ay!** *(Paramedic determines where the pain is located.)*
EMT	**¿Tiene vómitos y diarrea?**
Patient	**Sí.**
EMT	**¿Perdió el conocimiento?**
Patient	**No, pero estuve mareada.**
EMT	**No comprendo "mareada."**
Patient	*(Patient makes a hand gesture for "dizzy.")* **¿Entiende?**
EMT	**Sí, ¿Ha comido y bebido hoy?**
Patient	**Sí, agua.**
EMT	**¿Tiene una enfermedad crónica? ¿Diabetes? ¿Ulceras?**
Patient	**No, no.**
EMT	**Necesito tomarle el pulso y la presión.** *(Paramedic takes the patient's pulse and blood pressure.)* **Necesita líquidos. Vamos a ponerle un suero.**
Patient	**Está bien.**
EMT	**No se preocupe. ¿Qué hospital prefiere?**

Translation

EMT	**We're here to help. What's the problem?**
Patient	*(On the floor and very pale.)* **I fainted and I have a stomachache.**
EMT	**I don't understand. Does your stomach hurt?**
Patient	**Yes. I'm in a lot of pain.**
EMT	**Does it hurt here?**
Patient	**Yes, yes. Oh, oh!** *(Paramedic determines where the pain is located.)*
EMT	**Are you vomiting and have diarrhea?**
Patient	**Yes.**
EMT	**Did you lose consciousness?**
Patient	**No, but I was dizzy.**
EMT	**I don't understand "dizzy."**
Patient	*(Patient makes a hand gesture for "dizzy.")* **Understand?**
EMT	**Yes, did you eat or drink today?**
Patient	**Yes, water.**

(Continued on next page)

EMT	**Do you have a chronic illness? Diabetes? Ulcers?**
Patient	**No, no.**
EMT	**I need to take your pulse and blood pressure.** *(Paramedic takes the patient's pulse and blood pressure.)* **You need liquids. I'm going to start an IV.**
Patient	**OK.**
EMT	**Don't worry. What hospital do you prefer?**

AUDIO CD

III. Practice

Translate the following questions from English to Spanish. Repeat the exercise as often as you wish until you feel comfortable with your progress.

1. What's the problem? ______________________
2. Does it hurt here? ______________________
3. Do you have diarrhea? ______________________
4. Did you lose consciousness? ______________________
5. Did you eat or drink today? ______________________
6. What did you eat? ______________________
7. What did you drink? ______________________

AUDIO CD

Now let's practice a few of the phrases. Translate the following to Spanish.

1. I need to take your pulse. ______________________
2. Don't worry. ______________________
3. I'm going to start an IV. ______________________
4. I don't understand. ______________________
5. You need liquids. ______________________

For this exercise, you will be given a key word and you are to supply either the question or phrase that goes with it. There may be more than one possible answer so think of as many as you can. You might even come up with a few new ones.

1. Suero ______________________
   ____

2. Líquidos ______________________________

____

3. Estómago ______________________________

____

4. Conocimiento ______________________________

____

5. Diarrea y vómitos ______________________________

____

Provide the paramedic's lines for the following exchanges.

1. You: ______________________________

   Patient: Sí, me duele mucho el estómago.

2. You: ______________________________

   Patient: Sí, tengo diarrea y vómitos.

3. You: ______________________________

   Patient: ¿ Un suero? Ay, no, me duele.

4. You: ______________________________

   Patient: *(Extends his arm out for you to take vital signs.)*

5. You: ______________________________

   Patient: No importa, no tengo un hospital preferido.

AUDIO CD

IV. Vocabulary 2

Listen to the following vocabulary that was used by the patient in the dialogue. Remember that you wish to familiarize yourself with the words and phrases although you may not need to use them yourself.

Agua	Water
De	Of, from
Estómago	Stomach
Estoy	I am
Estuve	I was
Mareado(a)	Dizzy
Me desmayé.	I fainted.
Tengo dolor.	I have a pain.
Vomité.	I vomited.

Now you respond to the patient's statements and questions. There is more than one possible response and you will have to use phrases that you have learned in previous chapters.

1. Patient: Estoy mareado.

   You: ______________________________

2. Patient: Tengo dolor de estómago.

   You: ______________________________

3. Patient: Vomité mucho.

   You: ______________________________

4. Patient: Me desmayé.

   You: ______________________________

V. Review

Yes, it's time again to review and train your ear. Listen to the dialogue again. I'm sure it has become easier for you to understand the speakers. Of course, out in the field the people will be talking faster but you will find that with more and more exposure you'll be able to get the gist of what's going on. An excellent way to add to your exposure is simply by watching a little Spanish television if it's available in your area. If not, rent some Spanish movies with subtitles in English and see if you can pick up a few of the words. There are some good movies out there that will entertain you while training your ear. Have fun with it!

VI. Cultural Capsule

Religion

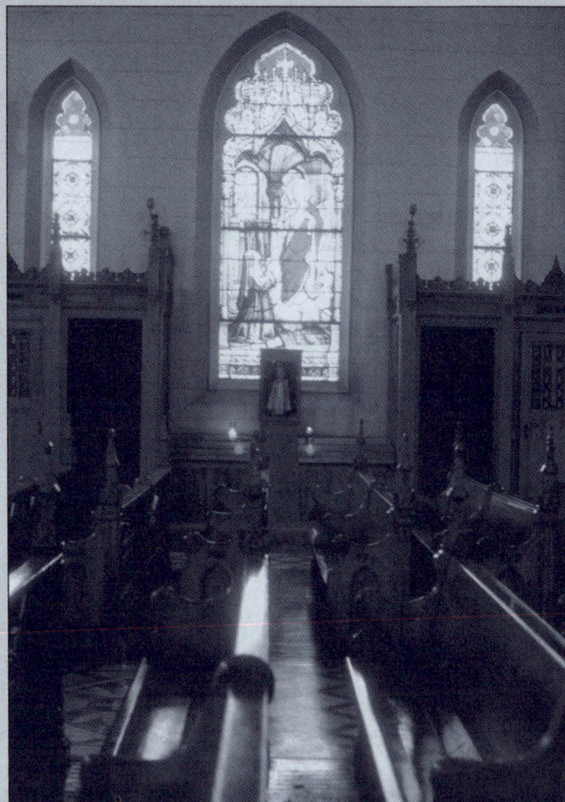

Religion plays an important role in the everyday life of many Hispanic and Latino people. It is an integral and evident part of their lives. Among Hispanics and Latinos, Catholicism is the main religion practiced. It is not unusual to go into someone's home and see signs of their faith, from crucifixes on the wall to altars bearing the picture of a patron saint. In an emergency situation, it is very common for the relatives to pray using their rosaries or to put religious objects on the patient to ensure his or her recovery. The much-used phrase of *"Dios mío,"* (My God), is not considered a curse in Spanish, but rather a means of asking for God's help or guidance. It is also possible that the patient or the family will wish to have a priest present at the hospital.

Co-existing with Catholicism are other "spiritual" and/or superstitious beliefs based on "Espiritismo" or "Santería." Although seen mainly in those from the Caribbean, healing practices based on these beliefs are seen throughout the Latin American population. Medics need to be aware that a "santero" or "curandero" (healer) may have been called to the scene or if the patient has been ill, one may have been consulted prior to calling 9-1-1. Some patients may believe that they have been victims of *"mal de ojo"* (the evil eye) and will need not only regular medical treatment but a charm, incantation, or potion from a "santero" in order to become completely cured.

Chapter 6

Illness 2: Cardiac Chest Pain

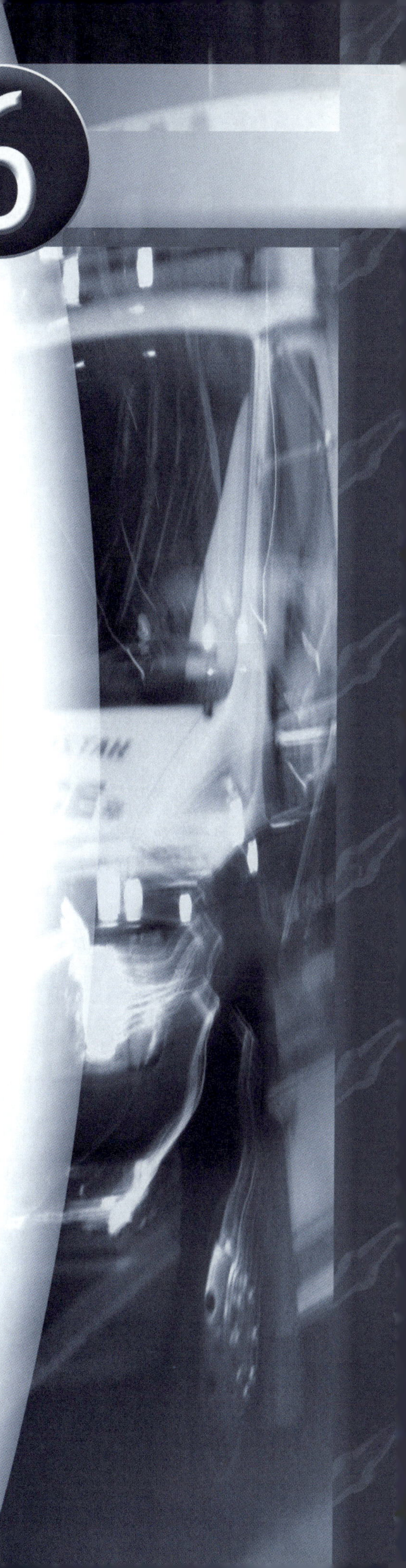

I. Vocabulary 1

AUDIO CD

Listen and repeat the following vocabulary. Always give yourself plenty of time and practice.

Commands

Señale dónde le duele.	Point to where it hurts.
Acuéstese en la camilla	Lay down on the stretcher.

Statements

Soy paramédico	I'm a paramedic.
Necesito ver la medicina.	I need to see the medicine.
Necesito tomarle el pulso y la presión.	I need to take your pulse and blood pressure.
Vamos al hospital.	We're going to the hospital.

Questions

¿Tiene náusea?	Are you nauseated? (Do you have nausea?)
¿Toma medicinas? ¿para el corazón?	Do you take medicines? for the heart?
¿Tomó la medicina hoy?	Did you take the medicine today?
¿Qué hospital prefiere?	What hospital do you prefer?

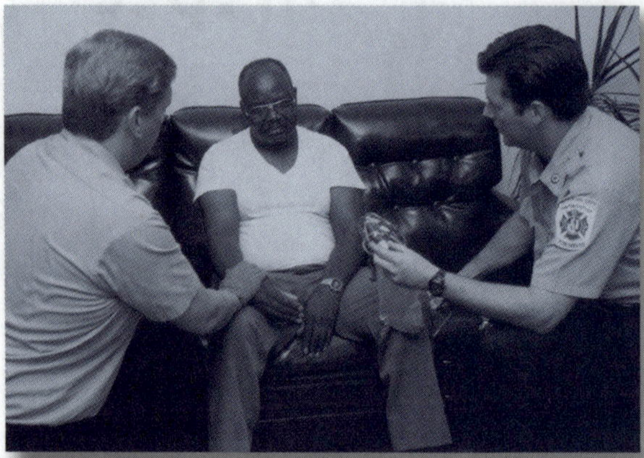

Translate the following using the Spanish vocabulary presented previously.

1. For the heart ______________
2. Lay down. ______________
3. The medicine ______________
4. I need ______________
5. On the stretcher ______________
6. Nauseated ______________
7. Do you have ______________
8. Point (to) ______________
9. Where it hurts ______________

Taking the phrases from the previous exercise, combine them to form four questions and/or phrases from the previous vocabulary. The sentences have been started for you.

1. Necesito tomarle ______________________________ .
2. Acuéstese en ______________________________ .
3. Señale dónde ______________________________ .
4. ¿Tiene ______________________________ ?

II. Dialogue

AUDIO CD

Listen to the following dialogue until you are able to understand it without reading it at the same time. It will take several sessions so don't give up too soon.

You arrive at a home where you find a man clutching his chest.

EMT	**Soy paramédico.**
Patient	**¡Ay! Me duele el pecho.** *(Clutches his chest.)*
EMT	**Señale dónde le duele.**

(Continued on next page)

Patient	Aquí. *(Points to chest and arm.)*
EMT	¿Tiene náusea?
Patient	Sí.
EMT	¿Toma medicinas para el corazón?
Patient	Sí. Digital.
EMT	¿Tomó la medicina hoy?
Patient	Sí.
EMT	Necesito ver la medicina.
Patient	Está allí, en la cocina. *(Someone brings the medicine from the kitchen.)*
EMT	Gracias. Acuéstese en la camilla, por favor. Necesito tomarle el pulso y la presión.
Patient	Está bien. *(EMT takes vital signs.)*
EMT	Vamos al hospital. ¿Qué hospital prefiere?
Patient	No importa.

Translation

EMT	I'm a paramedic.
Patient	Oh! My chest hurts! *(Clutches his chest.)*
EMT	Point to where it hurts.
Patient	Here. *(Points to chest and arm.)*
EMT	Are you nauseated?
Patient	Yes.
EMT	Do you take medicine for your heart?
Patient	Yes. Digitalis.
EMT	Did you take the medicine today?
Patient	Yes.
EMT	I need the medicine.
Patient	It's there, in the kitchen. *(Someone brings the medicine from the kitchen.)*
EMT	Thank you. Lay down on the stretcher, please. I need to take your pulse and blood pressure.
Patient	Ok. *(EMT takes vital signs.)*
EMT	We're going to the hospital. What hospital do you prefer?
Patient	It doesn't matter.

AUDIO CD

III. Practice

Translate the following from Spanish to English.

1. Acuéstese ______________________
2. La camilla ______________________
3. Para ______________________
4. El corazón ______________________
5. Aquí ______________________
6. Señale ______________________

7. Necesito ____________________
8. Vamos ____________________
9. Dónde ____________________
10. Me duele ____________________
11. Toma ____________________
12. La medicina ____________________
13. Paramédico ____________________
14. Bien ____________________
15. Al hospital ____________________

AUDIO CD

Translate the following phrases from English to Spanish. You will be building the phrases backward from end to beginning and then saying the completed question or statement. Become comfortable with these expressions.

1. to the hospital, we're going — We're going to the hospital.

   ____

2. (do you) prefer, what hospital — What hospital do you prefer?

   ____

3. on the stretcher, lay down — Lay down on the stretcher.

   ____

4. for the heart, medicine, do you take — Do you take medicine for the heart?

   ____

5. today, the medicine, did you take — Did you take the medicine today?

   ____

6. nausea, do you have — Do you have nausea? (Are you nauseated?)

   ____

What phrases or questions might you employ in the following situations?

1. You need to know what medicine the patient is taking. ____________________

   ____

2. You want to know where the medicine is. ____________________

   ____

3. You want to know where it hurts. ____________________

   ____

4. You want to know if the patient has taken any medicine today. ______________

____

5. You need for the patient to lay down on the stretcher. ______________

____

AUDIO CD

IV. Vocabulary 2

Repeat the following vocabulary and become familiar with it. Try to remember how the words were combined in the dialogue presented previously. Also think of situations in which you might have heard these spoken before. Always relate the words to yourself and how you might use them.

Me duele	________ hurts me
El pecho	The chest
La digital	The digitalis
Está allí	It's there
En la cocina	In the kitchen
No importa	It's not important

Respond to the patient's comments.

1. You: ______________________________________

   Patient: Sí, me duele mucho el pecho.

2. You: ______________________________________

   Patient: La medicina está allí.

3. You: ______________________________________

   Patient: Sí, tomo digital.

4. You: ______________________________________

   Patient: ¿El hospital? No importa.

V. Review

You're doing a great job! Go back and review by listening to the dialogue again. Remember to write down the questions and phrases that you find useful on cards and keep practicing.

VI. Cultural Capsule

Motherhood

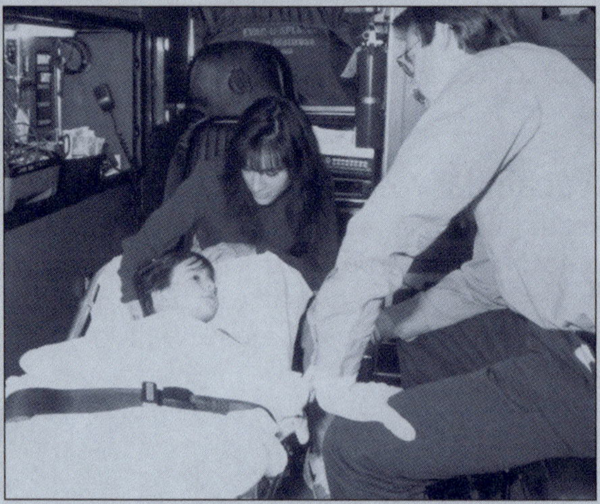

Just as in many other communities, within the Hispanic community, being a mother is considered a woman's most important role in life. She is the one who supports her family through emotional, as well as, physical trauma. She is sacred to her children and is loved and respected for the unconditional care that she gives.

For the health provider, this is important to know because of the great attachment that exists between a mother and her children. She has been their doctor and nurse and will not wish to be separated from them when they are hurt or ill. Although it is not so different from non-Hispanic cultures, one must take into account the cultural and language barriers that add to the children's and the mother's anxiety in being separated, particularly in traumatic situations. A mother may become quite upset if her child is seriously hurt, but will calm down if there is something that she can do to help. Simply by allowing her to hold her child's hand or stroke his brow may be enough to calm her and enable her to give support to an ill or injured child.

Chapter 7

Having a Baby

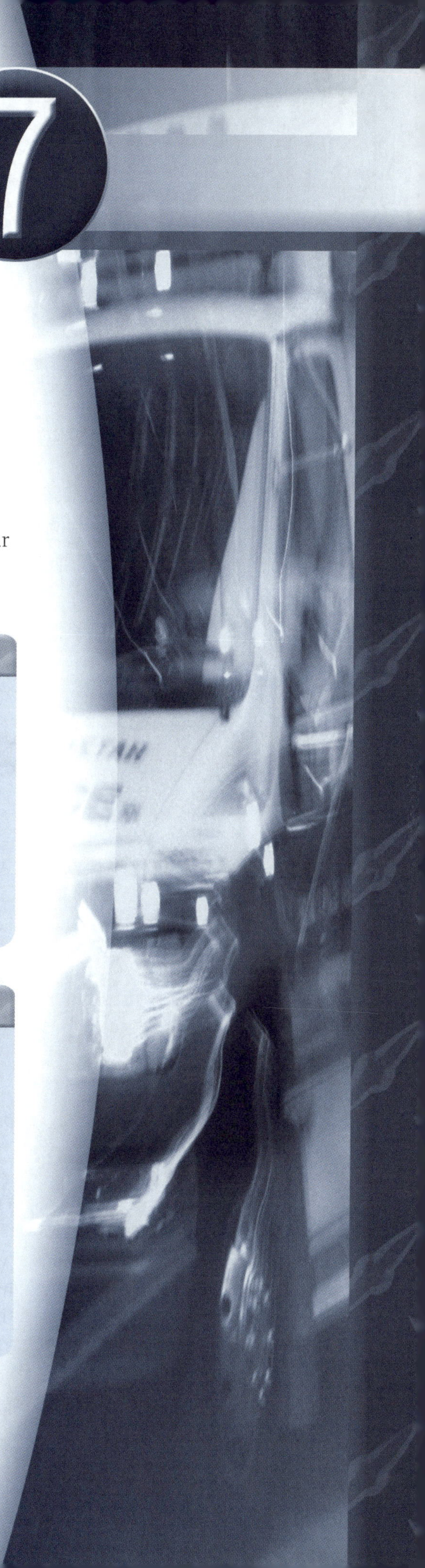

I. Vocabulary 1

AUDIO CD

The following vocabulary should help you deal with gynecologic situations. Again, repeat after the speaker until you are comfortable with your pronunciation and understanding of the phrases. Always remember, especially with commands, to use *por favor.* ¡Buena suerte!

Commands

Acuéstese	Lay down
Empuje	Push
No empuje	Don't push
Espere	Wait
No se preocupe	Don't worry
Dígame	Tell me
Cuándo le duele	When it hurts
Respire	Breathe

Statements

Es un varón.	It's a boy.
Es una hembra.	It's a girl.
Vamos a ayudar.	We're going to help you.
Necesito examinarla.	I need to examine you.
Yo espero.	I'll wait/I hope.
Aquí tiene su bebé.	Here is your baby.
Es la placenta.	It's the placenta.
Todo está bien.	Everything is fine.
Tengo que cortar	I have to cut
El cordón umbilical	The umbilical cord

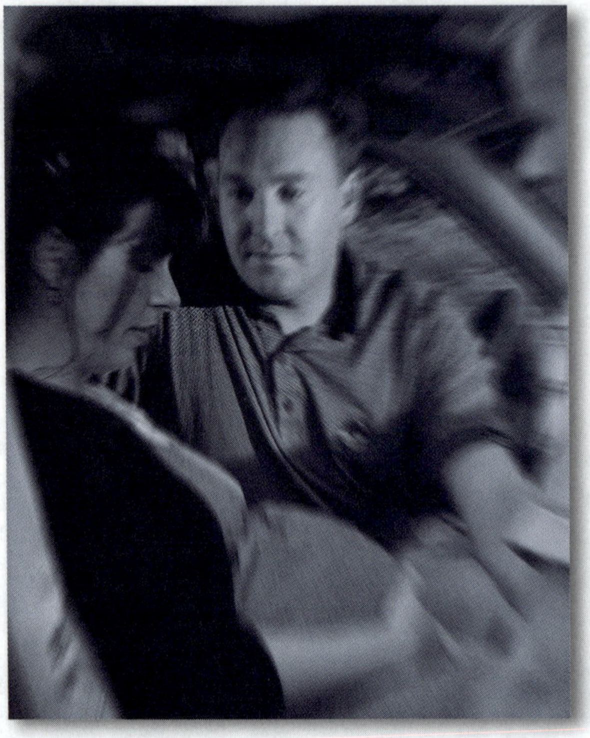

Questions

¿Está embarazada? ¿Está en estado?	Are you pregnant?
¿Está a punto de dar a luz?	Are you about to give birth?
¿A cuántos minutos están los dolores?	How many minutes apart are the pains?
¿Cuántos meses tiene de embarazo?	How many months pregnant are you?
¿Es su primer bebé?	Is this your first baby?
¿Fue un parto natural?	Did you have the baby naturally?
¿Tuvo complicaciones antes?	Did you have any complications before?
¿Tiene complicaciones con este bebé?	Do you have any complications with this baby?
¿Tuvo una cesárea antes?	Did you have a cesarean before?
¿Ya se le rompió la fuente?	Did your water break already?

After you have listened to the above sentences, continue to the following individual words and phrases. You may wish to practice these several times. You'll be amazed at how much more you'll understand the more you practice.

1. Ahora ______
2. Antes ______
3. Bebé ______
4. Dolores ______
5. Cesárea ______
6. Complicaciones ______
7. Embarazada ______
8. Examinarla ______
9. Fuente ______
10. Ombligo ______
11. Cordón umbilical ______
12. Se rompió ______
13. Todo ______

We're going to do one more exercise before moving on to the dialogue. Check out the following situations and write the appropriate Spanish response.

1. A woman is complaining of pain in her lower abdomen and you wish to determine if she is pregnant. ______
2. You wish to know how many months pregnant she is. ______
3. You wish to know if she's had other children. ______
4. You want to reassure her and her family. ______
5. You need to tell her not to push yet. ______

AUDIO CD

II. Dialogue

Medic enters the home of a Hispanic family and finds that no one speaks English and the mother is about to have a baby. The mother is sitting up on the sofa.

EMT	**Vamos a ayudar. No se preocupe.**
Patient	**¡Ay cómo me duele!**
EMT	**¿Está embarazada? ¿Está a punto de dar a luz?**
Patient	**Sí, me duele mucho.**
EMT	**¿A cuántos minutos están los dolores?**
Patient	**No sé, quizás cada tres minutos.**

(Continued on next page)

EMT **¿Cuánto duran los dolores?**

Patient **Un minuto.**

EMT **¿Cuántos meses tiene de embarazo?**

Patient **Ocho y medio.**

EMT **¿Es su primer bebé?**

Patient **No, es mi tercero.**

EMT **¿Fueron partos naturales?**

Patient **Sí.**

EMT **¿Tuvo complicaciones o una cesárea antes?**

Patient **No. ¡Ay cómo me duele!**

EMT **¿Ya se le rompió la fuente?**

Patient **Sí. ¡Ay, cómo me duele!** *(EMT waits for the contraction to be over.)*

EMT **Por favor, necesito examinarla. No se preocupe. Acuéstese, por favor.**

Patient **Está bien. ¿y los dolores?**

EMT **Dígame cuando le duele y yo espero.**

Patient **¡Ay! Ya me empieza. Quiero empujar.**

EMT **Por favor respire lentamente por la boca.** *(Determines that patient may push.)* **Bien, ahora empuje, señora.**

Patient **Aquí viene el bebé.** *(Baby is delivered. EMT clears the airway, wraps baby, cuts the cord and gives him to the mother.)*

EMT **Es un varón. Todo está bien. Tengo que cortar el cordón umbilical. Aquí tiene el bebé, señora.**

Patient **Gracias...** *(Mother and baby are taken to the ambulance. On the way to the hospital the mother begins to deliver the placenta.)* **¡Aquí viene otro dolor!**

EMT **Sí, señora, es la placenta. Por favor, empuje.** *(The placenta is delivered. Mom and baby are fine.)* **Todo está bien.**

Translation

EMT **We're going to help. Don't worry.**

Patient **Oh, it hurts!**

EMT **Are you pregnant? Are you about to give birth?**

Patient **Yes, it hurts a lot.**

EMT **How many minutes apart are the pains** *(contractions)***?**

Patient **I don't know. Maybe three minutes.**

EMT **How long do the pains last?**

Patient **About a minute.**

EMT **How many months pregnant are you?**

Patient **8 ½.**

EMT **Is this your first baby?**

Patient **No, it's my third.**

EMT **Did you have the babies naturally?**

Patient **Yes.**

EMT **Did you have complications or a cesarean before?**

Patient **No. Oh, how it hurts.**

(Continued on next page)

EMT	**Did your water break?**
Patient	**Yes. Oh, it really hurts.** *(EMT waits for the contraction to be over.)*
EMT	**Please, I need to examine you. Don't worry. Please lay down.**
Patient	**Fine, and the pains?**
EMT	**Tell me when you are in pain and I'll wait.**
Patient	**Oh, it's beginning. I want to push.**
EMT	**Please breathe slowly through your mouth.** *(Determines that the patient may push.)* **Ok, now push, ma'am.**
Patient	**Here comes the baby.** *(Baby is delivered. EMT clears the airway, cuts the cord, and gives him to the mother.)*
EMT	**It's a boy. Everything is fine. I have to cut the cord. Here is your baby.**
Patient	**Thank you.** *(Mother and baby are taken to the ambulance. On the way to the hospital the mother begins to deliver the placenta.)* **Here comes another pain.**
EMT	**Yes, ma'am. That's the placenta. Please push.** *(The placenta is delivered. Mom and baby are fine.)* **Everything is fine.**

AUDIO CD

III. Practice

Repeat the following words and translate to the English.

1. Empuje ______________________
2. Varón ______________________
3. Hembra ______________________
4. Fuente ______________________
5. Bebé ______________________
6. Dígame ______________________
7. Dolores ______________________
8. Primer ______________________
9. Respire ______________________
10. Lentamente ______________________

AUDIO CD

Repeat the following questions in Spanish and translate to English. Remember to do this exercise as many times as you wish until you are comfortable with these questions.

1. ¿Está a punto de dar a luz ahora? ______________________
2. ¿A cuántos minutos están los dolores ahora? ______________________
3. ¿Ya se le rompió la fuente? ______________________
4. ¿Tuvo complicaciones antes? ______________________
5. ¿Cuántos meses tiene de embarazo? ______________________
6. ¿A cuántos minutos están los dolores? ______________________

What would you say in the following situations?

1. You wish to know how many months pregnant the woman is. ______________________

2. You wish to examine a woman who is a bit nervous. ______________________

3. You need for the woman to push. ______________________

4. It's the woman's first baby and she doesn't know that the placenta must also be delivered. ______________________

5. You wish to tell the woman that she has a baby girl. ______________________

AUDIO CD

Translate the following questions to Spanish. Remember to repeat the answers and to do the exercise as often as you like.

1. Are you pregnant? ______________________
2. How many months pregnant are you? ______________________
3. How many minutes apart are the pains? ______________________
4. Is this your first baby? ______________________
5. Has your water broken? ______________________
6. Did you have any complications before? ______________________
7. Please push. ______________________
8. Breathe. ______________________
9. I have to cut the cord. ______________________
10. You have a baby boy. ______________________

IV. Vocabulary 2

AUDIO CD

Now you will hear some phrases that might be said by the patient or bystanders. For this vocabulary, remember that, except for the numbers, it is more important that you understand rather than duplicate. Listen and repeat.

STATEMENTS

¡Ay cómo me duele!	Oh, how it hurts!
¡Me duele mucho!	It hurts a lot!
No sé.	I don't know.
Cada tres minutos.	Every three minutes.
Ya me empieza el dolor.	The pain (contraction) is beginning.
Quiero empujar.	I want to push.

ORDINAL NUMBERS

primero	first	sexto	sixth
segundo	second	séptimo	seventh
tercero	third	octavo	eighth
cuarto	fourth	noveno	ninth
quinto	fifth	décimo	tenth

NUMBERS

uno	one	seis	six
dos	two	siete	seven
tres	three	ocho	eight
cuatro	four	nueve	nine
cinco	five	diez	ten

AUDIO CD

Say in English what the woman is saying in Spanish. Listen to the statements as often as you wish until you become familiar with them.

1. No sé. ____________________
2. Quiero empujar. ____________________
3. ¡Ay cómo me duele! ____________________
4. Ya me empieza el dolor. ____________________
5. ¡Me duele mucho! ____________________

In this exercise you will need to write down the number that the patient says when asked, "*¿Cuántos meses tiene de embarazo?*"

1. ______________________ 4. ______________________

2. ______________________ 5. ______________________

3. ______________________ 6. ______________________

Now you will hear the question, "*¿A cuántos minutos están los dolores?*" Write down the numerical response of the patient. You need to listen carefully since the patient may add to the information that you are seeking.

1. ______________________ 4. ______________________

2. ______________________ 5. ______________________

3. ______________________

It is possible that a patient will answer using the ordinal numbers for a question such as, "*¿Es su primer hijo?*" For this exercise write down the ordinal number that you hear when a patient is asked the above question.

1. ______________________ 6. ______________________

2. ______________________ 7. ______________________

3. ______________________ 8. ______________________

4. ______________________ 9. ______________________

5. ______________________ 10. ______________________

V. Review

Great! You've finished one of the most difficult chapters of this book and should be feeling pretty good about all the work you've done. Now, we'll do a quick review. You'll be given the situation and you need to provide the commands, statements, or questions that you might use. Remember that at times there is more than one possibility.

1. A woman is complaining of abdominal pains and you cannot tell that she is pregnant from simply looking at her. ______________________

____

2. You wish to know if she had any other babies before and if she had any complications. ______________________

____

3. You need to examine her and reassure her at the same time. ______________________________

4. You need to tell her to breathe slowly and push. ______________________________

5. You need to tell the woman that you need to cut the cord. ______________________________

VI. Cultural Capsule

Fathers and Childbirth

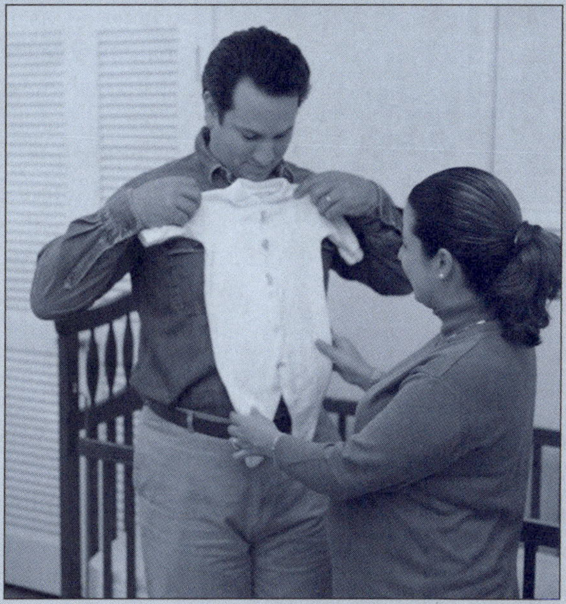

In many parts of the Latino world, childbirth is still considered to be a woman's sole domain. Many fathers are comfortable not being present during childbirth. Indeed, they may find it quite embarrassing to be present while their wives are giving birth, especially if there are other women present. It is not uncommon for some fathers to be helpless bystanders in such situations.

For the medic, it is important to recognize this and to be aware of the father's possible reaction should his wife go into labor before reaching the hospital. If the father has not participated in birthing classes, he may be reluctant to help for fear of causing injury to the mother or the infant. The mother may actually prefer the presence of another woman over that of her husband. Although the role of the father in childbirth is changing, the medic may still encounter this situation in the field.

Chapter 8

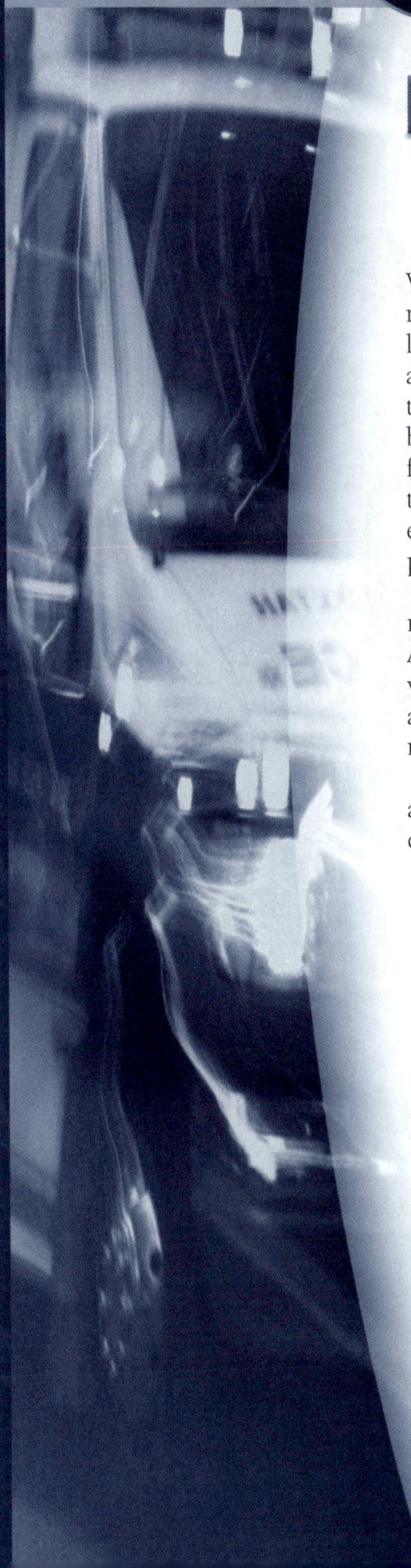

Review

Well, you have survived the course and you should be proud of having mastered the material presented. Learning even a small bit of another language is a challenging and hopefully rewarding experience. It is an admirable endeavor to wish to communicate more easily with others at a time when so many are alienated in their lives. This course is only a beginning. It will help you to bridge the gap but it will be you out in the field helping and communicating with your patients that will truly make the difference. You will find that the more you try out the language the easier it will get and the more you will begin to pick up from your patients. So, as I said earlier, this course is only a beginning.

Now, it is time again for you to design your own set of questions and responses based on your experience. You may wish to refer to Appendix A as a guide. What questions will be helpful to you as you deal with the varying illnesses that you encounter every day? What words of reassurance will you be likely to need in order to calm a patient or a family member? Write these down and practice them until you are satisfied.

Remember to keep it fun by listening to music, watching TV or movies and, if at all possible, find someone to talk to in Spanish. Language is for communication so… keep communicating!

Appendix A

Controlling and Assessing the Scene

Below are most of the phrases and questions that you will need in controlling a scene and in assessing the patient's condition. The phrases have been divided into "key verbs," "commands," "questions," and "other expressions." You will want to repeat these to review what you have already learned. Later you may want to use this section simply as a reference.

Key Verbs

As you progressed through the book you may have noticed that these "key verbs" are used constantly in phrases and questions. It is a good idea to memorize them individually so they will be readily available to you on any occasion.

Es (soy)	Is, (I am)
Está	Is, (location, condition)
Le duele	_________ hurts you/him/her
Me duele	_________ hurts me
Me oye?	Do you hear me?
Necesita	You/he/she needs
Necesito	I need
Perdió	Did you lose
Prefiere	You/he/she prefers
Prefiero	I prefer
Tiene	You have, he/she has
Tengo	I have
Tomó	Did you take or drink
Voy a	I am going to
Vamos	We're going (let's go).

Commands

Acuéstese	Lay down
Señale	Point
Cálmese	Calm down
Siéntese	Sit down
Déme	Give me
Silencio	Silence
Escriba	Write
Vaya	Go
Empuje	Push
Levántese	Get up, stand up
Venga	Come
No se levante	Don't get up
Mire	Look
Míreme	Look at me
Mire para arriba	Look up
Muévase	Move
No se mueva	Don't move

Questions 1

Questions: Sí/No

Assessing the symptoms (Los síntomas)

The following questions are based on symptoms and at times use colloquial expressions for body parts or illnesses. Most have been used in the text and, hopefully, you are familiar with them. You will note that the verb ***tiene*** (do you have) is the key to asking many of these yes/no questions. You may wish to practice these by repeating and doing exercises similar to the ones that you have done throughout the book. Get some index cards and write down the categories on one side and the questions on the other. Practice until you can ask the questions without too much effort. Go back and repeat the correct pronunciation until you're satisfied with your utterances.

General symptoms

Does ________ hurt?	¿Le duele ________ ?
Do you have any pain?	¿Tiene dolor?
Do you feel weak?	¿Tiene debilidad? ¿Se siente débil?
Do you have a fever?	¿Tiene fiebre?
Do you have chills?	¿Tiene escalofríos?
Are you dizzy?	¿Está mareado(a)?
Are you bleeding?	¿Está sangrando?

Skin-related (la piel)

Do you have a rash?	¿Tiene erupciones en la piel?
Do you itch?	¿Tiene picazón?
Are you swollen?	¿Está hinchado?
Were you stung by an insect?	¿Lo picó un insecto (bicho)?
Were you bitten by a spider?	¿Lo picó una araña?

Bleeding and/or bruises

Do you have a bruise?	¿Tiene un morado (moretón)?
Are you bleeding?	¿Está sangrando?
Do you have a wound?	¿Tiene una herida?
Were you bitten by an animal?	¿Lo mordió un animal?

Eyes and ears

Do you have blurred vision?	¿Tiene la visión borrosa?
Do you hear a buzzing noise?	¿Oye un zumbido?
Can you hear me?	¿Me oye?
Do you have an earache?	¿Tiene dolor de oído?

Nose and throat

Do you have a bloody nose?	¿Tiene sangre por la nariz?
Are you congested?	¿Tiene congestión nasal?
Do you have trouble breathing?	¿Tiene dificultad al respirar?
Are you coughing?	¿Tiene tos?
Do you have asthma?	¿Tiene asma?
Do you have allergies?	¿Tiene alergias?

Neurologic

Do you have a headache?	¿Tiene dolor de cabeza? ¿Le duele la cabeza?
Do you have double vision?	¿Ve doble?
Do you have loss of sensation?	¿Tiene falta de sensación?
Did you lose consciousness?	¿Perdió el conocimiento?

Cardiovascular

Do you have chest pain?	¿Tiene dolor de pecho?
Do you have palpitations?	¿Tiene palpitaciones?

Gastrointestinal

Do you have a stomachache?	¿Tiene dolor de estómago?
Do you have nausea?	¿Tiene náusea?
Have you been vomiting?	¿Tiene vómitos?
Do you have blood in the vomit?	¿Tiene sangre en el vómito?
Do you have blood in your stool?	¿Tiene sangre en las materias fecales?
Do you have diarrhea?	¿Tiene diarrea?
Do you have constipation?	¿Tiene estreñimiento?

Genitourinary

Do you have difficulty urinating?	¿Tiene dificultad al orinar?
Do you have pain?	¿Tiene dolor?

Pregnancy

Are you pregnant?	¿Está embarazada?
Are you in pain?	¿Tiene dolor?
Are you having the baby now?	¿Está a punto de dar a luz?

Muscles and joints

Do you have muscle pain?	¿Tiene dolores musculares?
Do you have a backache?	¿Tiene dolor de espalda?
Do you have joint pain?	¿Tiene dolores de articulación?
Do you have any swelling?	¿Tiene hinchazón?
Are you fatigued?	¿Tiene fatiga?

Poison and drugs

Did you take a medicine or drug?	¿Tomó alguna medicina o drogas?
Did you take poison? What?	¿Tomó algún veneno? ¿Qué?
Did you vomit?	¿Vomitó?

Bites and stings

Were you bitten by an animal?	¿Lo mordió un animal?
a dog?	¿un perro?
a cat?	¿un gato?
a snake?	¿una serpiente?
a wild animal?	¿un animal salvaje?
Were you stung by an insect?	¿Lo picó un insecto (bicho)?
a spider?	¿una araña?

Pain

Do you have any pain?	¿Tiene dolor?
Does ________ hurt?	¿Le duele ________ ?
Is the pain strong?	¿Es el dolor fuerte
weak?	leve?
moderate?	moderado?
sharp?	agudo?
stabbing?	punzante?
constant?	constante?
Does the pain radiate?	¿Se extiende el dolor?

Medical history

Do you have allergies to medicines?	¿Tiene alergias a alguna medicina?
Do you suffer from an illness?	¿Tiene una enfermedad?**
Do you have problems with your heart?	¿Tiene problemas con el corazón?
diabetes?	la diabetes?
blood pressure?	la presión?
breathing?	la respiración
Did you have an accident today?	¿Tuvo un accidente hoy?

*** Please note that a list of illnesses using both standard and colloquial Spanish has been provided in Appendix B.*

Questions 2

Information

The following questions will elicit information from the patient. These are not "yes or no" questions. Therefore, the Spanish speaker may ramble on and you may not be able to follow. Always be prepared with the phrase "No comprendo," (*I don't understand*) or "más despacio, por favor," (*slower, please*).

Basic questions

¿Cuándo?	When?	¿Qué?	What?
¿Dónde?	Where?	¿.Quién?	Who?

Information

¿Cuándo ocurrió?	When did it happen?
¿Dónde está el cuchillo?	Where is the knife?
¿Dónde está la pistola?	Where is the gun?
¿Dónde le duele?	Where does it hurt?
¿Qué hospital prefiere?	What hospital do you prefer?
¿Qué problema tiene?	What's the problem?
¿Quién es el paciente?	Who is the patient?
¿Quién necesita ayuda?	Who needs help?
¿Su nombre?	Your name?
¿Su dirección?	Your address?
¿Su número de teléfono?	Your telephone number?
¿Su seguro?	Your insurance?
¿Su número de seguro social?	Your Social Security number?
¿Su licencia?	Your license?

Other Expressions

Below, you will find a list of other helpful expressions that you practiced throughout this program.

Gracias	Thank you
Por favor	Please
Sí	Yes
No	No
No comprendo.	I don't understand.
Necesito.	I need.
Más despacio	Slower
Soy paramédico.	I'm a paramedic.
Tomarle el pulso/la presión	Take your pulse/blood pressure
Vamos a ayudar.	We're going to help.

Appendix B

Illnesses

English	Spanish (standard and colloquial)
AIDS	SIDA
Allergies	Alergias
Appendicitis	Apendicitis, apendis
Arthritis	Artritis, reuma
Asthma	Asma, ahogo, mal de pecho
Bite	Mordedura, mordida
Bronchitis	Bronquitis
Burns	Quemaduras, quemadas
Cancer	Cáncer
Chicken pox	Varicela, viruelas locas, peste cristal
Congestion	Constipado, congestión, estar tupido
Convulsions	Convulsiones, ataques, tiritones
Cold	Resfriado, catarro, gripe, enfriamiento
Cough	Tos
Diabetes	Diabetes
Epileptic seizure	Ataque de epilepsia
Fever	Fiebre
Flu	Influenza, gripe, gripa
Fractures	Fractura, huesos quebrados (rotos)
Headache	Dolor de cabeza, la jaqueca
Heart attack	Infarto del corazón, ataque, mal del corazón
Hepatitis	Hepatitis
Hernia	Hernia, rotura, desaldillado
Hypertension	Hipertensión, presión arterial alta, presión alta, tensión alta
Infection	Infección de ________
Measles	Sarampión, alfombrilla

(Continued on next page)

English	Spanish (standard and colloquial)
Meningitis	Meningitis
Mucus	Moco(s)
Parasites	Parásitos, parasitosis, gusanos (animalitos), lombrices, bichos
Pneumonia	Pulmonía, neumonía
Poisoning	El envenenamiento, la intoxicación
Poliomyelitis	Poliomielitis, polio, parálisis infantil
Rheumatism	Reumatismo, reuma
Sinusitis	Sinusitis
Smallpox	Viruela
Sneeze	Estomudar
Sting	Picadura, picada, piquete
Sunstroke	Insolación, asoleada, golpe de calor, mucho sol
Tetanus	Tétano
Tuberculosis	Tuberculosis, tísico, tisis, tis
Ulcers	Ulceras, dolor de aire, empacho
Urinary infection	Infección urinaria, mal de orín(a)
Venereal disease	Enfermedad venérea, secreta

Appendix C

Colloquial Expressions for Parts of the Body

There are many different groups of Hispanics living in the United States. At times, the vocabulary used by one national group may be different from that used by another. Because of this, you should be aware of where the majority of your patients are from and get to know the specific vocabulary that you will need to work efficiently with the community. The basic vocabulary presented in this book is what is considered "standard" and will be understood by any Spanish speaker. Below, however, is a list of colloquial expressions for different body parts that you may hear from your patients. It is the equivalent of calling a "stomach" a "gut." It is my fervent wish that this list will be helpful in allowing you to assess your patients more precisely.

English	Standard	Colloquial
Abdomen	El abdomen	El estómago, la panza, la barriga
Ankle	El tobillo	
Appendix	El apéndice	El apendis
Back	La espalda	El espinazo, el lomo
Bladder	La vejiga	
Blood	La sangre	El coco, la pupa
Bone	El hueso	
Brain	El cerebro	Los sesos, el coco
Breast	El seno	Los pechos, las chichis, las tetas, las mamas
Breastbone	El esternón	El hueso del pecho
Buttocks	Las nalgas	El fondillo, el culo, la cola, las sentaderas, el pompis
Chest	El torax	El pecho
Collarbone	La clavícula	El hueso del cuello
Colon	El colon	El intestino mayor
Complexion	El cutis	La piel
Crotch	La ingle	La entrepierna

(Continued on next page)

English	Standard	Colloquial
Esophagus	El esófago	El tragante, la boca del estómago, el gaznate
Eye	El ojo	La vista
Face	La cara	El rostro
Gallbladder	La vesícula	La hiel
Genitals	Los genitales	Las partes, el entresijo
Groin	La ingle	El entresijo, la aldilla
Hair	El pelo	El cabello, las greñas
Body hair	El vello	
Pubic hair	El vello púbico, pelo del pubis	El pendejo
Head	La cabeza	La chompeta, el coco
Hip	La cadera	El cuadril
Intestine	El intestino	La tripa
Jaw	La mandíbula	La quijada
Joint	La articulación	La coyuntura
Liver	El hígado	
Mouth	La boca	La trompa, el hocico
Nail	La uña	La garra, la pezuña
Neck	El cuello, la nuca	El pescuezo
Penis	El pene	El palo, el falo, el miembro la cosa, el chile, el pito, etc.
Prostate gland	La próstata	La glándula masculina
Rectum	El recto	El ano, el culo, el trasero
Ribs	Las costillas	
Side	El lado	El costado, el ijar, la ijada
Skeleton	El esqueleto	Los huesos
Skin	La piel	El pellejo, la carne
Skull	El cráneo	La calavera
Stomach	El estómago	La panza, la barriga
Throat	La garganta	El tragadero
Trachea	La tráquea	El gaznate
Vertebra	La vértebra	Los huesos, el espinazo
Waist	La cintura	El talle, la espalda (back)

Appendix D

Numbers

You may need to become familiar with the numbers in Spanish in order to determine when something happened.

Numbers 1 - 20; 30 - 100 (by tens)

1 uno	11 once	30 treinta
2 dos	12 doce	40 cuarenta
3 tres	13 trece	50 cincuenta
4 cuatro	14 catorce	60 sesenta
5 cinco	15 quince	70 setenta
6 seis	16 dieciséis	80 ochenta
7 siete	17 diecisiete	90 noventa
8 ocho	18 dieciocho	100 cien
9 nueve	19 diecinueve	
10 diez	20 veinte	

Telling Time

When you wish to know when something happened the phrase is, "¿A qué hora ocurrió?" or "¿Cuándo ocurrió?" *(When did it happen?)*. The person may answer, "A las dos," meaning, *"At two,"* or it is possible to answer that it happened so many minutes or hours ago. In this case, the phrase is, "Hace dos horas," meaning, *"Two hours ago."* Literally the phrase in Spanish means, "It makes two hours." Now, study the following examples and then see if you can formulate the questions and answers on your own.

Examples:

¿A qué hora ocurrió? A las tres.

¿Cuándo ocurrió? Hace 20 minutos.

Practice:

1. When did it happen? At two.

____

2. When did it happen? It was four hours ago.

____

3. When did it happen? At five.

____

4. When did it happen? It was six hours ago.

____

5. When did it happen? At ten.

____

Appendix E

Family Relationships

The vocabulary presented here may be helpful to you when dealing with the family members. You will notice that some of the words end in either an "o" or an "a." The "o" endings designate that the person is male and the "a" ending designates female.

A Large Family	
Esposo (a)	Husband (wife)
Abuelo (a)	Grandfather (grandmother)
Madre (Mamá, Mami)	Mother
Padre (Papá, Papi)	Father
Hijo	Son
Hija	Daughter
Hermano	Brother
Hermana	Sister
Bebé	Baby
Tío	Uncle
Tía	Aunt
Novio	Boyfriend
Novia	Girlfriend
Amigo (a)	Friend

As you are dealing with the people at the scene, you may need to ask who someone is, "¿Quién es él (he)?" or "¿Quién es ella (she)?" What are some other questions that you might ask concerning the people around the patient?

Appendix F

Insurance Form

Below, you will find translations of terms that should help in preparing the paperwork you will need to fill out for your patients.

Name	Nombre
Street Address	Dirección (Domicilio)
Apartment Number	Número de apartamento
City	Ciudad
County	Condado
Zip Code	Zip Code (código postal)
Home Telephone	Número de teléfono de su casa
Work Telephone	Número de teléfono de su trabajo
Employer	Empleado por
Social Security Number	Número de Seguro Social
Insurance Company	Compañía de Seguro Médico
Group Number	Número del grupo del Seguro
Individual Identification Number	Número individual del Seguro
Date of Birth	Fecha de nacimiento
Nearest Relative	Pariente más cercano

Appendix G

Equipment List

English	Español
Cot	Camilla
Blanket	Frazada/ Manta/ Cobija
Seat Belt	Cinturón de seguridad
Oxygen	Oxígeno
Oxygen Mask	Máscara de oxígeno
Nasal Cannula	Cánula nasal
Oxygen Treatment	Tratamiento de oxígeno
Oral Airway	Vía aérea oral
Nasal Airway	Vía aérea nasal
Endotrachael Tube	Tubo endotraqueal
Laryngoscope	Laringoscopía
Intravenous Fluid	Líquidos intravenosos
Catheter	Catéter/Sonda
Tourniquet	Torniquete
Syringe	Jeringa/Jeringuilla
Medication	Medicamento/Medicina
Defibrillator	Desfibrilador
Cardiac Monitor	Monitor cardiaco
Electrodes	Electrodos
Glucometer	Glucómetro
Backboard	Tabla para la espalda
Cervical Collar	Collar cervical
Straps	Correas/Tiras
Dressing	Venda/Vendaje
Splint	Férula/Tablilla
Traction Splint	Tablilla de tracción
KED (Kendricks Extrication Device)	Máquina de extraer de Kendricks
Portable Stretcher	Camilla portátil
Bag Mask	Máscara
Thumper (Mechanical CPR device)	Máquina de golpe torácico

Answers

to Exercise Questions

Chapter 1

Page 2

I. 1. a, b, c 2. b, c 3. a 4. a, b

Pages 4-5

III. 1. Silence, please. 2. I have questions. 3. Slower. 4. We're going to help. 5. Calm down. 6. Sit down. 7. Don't worry. 8. I don't understand. 9. A lot or a little 10. Who needs help? 11. I'm a paramedic. 12. I speak a little Spanish. 13. Are you the mother?

Page 5

1. Un poco 2. De español 3. Hablo 4. Ayuda. 5. Necesita 6. Quién 7. Ayudarle 8. Vamos a 9. Un paramédico 10. Soy 11. Por favor 12. Siéntese.

Page 5

1. Hablo un poco de español. 2. ¿Quién necesita ayuda? 3. Vamos a ayudarle. 4. Soy un paramédico. 5. Siéntese, por favor.

Pages 5-6

1. No comprendo. 2. Hablo un poco de español. 3. Cálmese. 4. Más despacio, por favor. 5. No se preocupe. 6. ¿Quién necesita ayuda? 7. Soy un paramédico. 8. Vamos a ayudarle. 9. Siéntese, por favor. 10. ¿Mucho o poco? 11. Tengo unas preguntas. 12. Silencio, por favor.

Page 6

1. Vamos a ayudarle. Soy un paramédico. 2. ¿Le duele mucho o poco? 3. Cálmese. Siéntese. 4. No comprendo. Tengo unas preguntas.

Page 7

IV. 1. Oh, I'm in a lot of pain. 2. It hurts here. 3. Oh, no! It's bleeding a lot. 4. How painful! Help me! 5. He is vomiting. He has the flu.

Chapter 2

Page 10

I. 1. ¿Cómo ocurrió? 2. ¿Dónde le duele? 3. ¿Cuándo ocurrió?

Page 11

1. Point. Point to where it hurts. 2. Calm down. Calm down, please. 3. Sit down. Sit down here, please. 4. Look. Look up. Look at me.

Page 11

1. Necesito tomarle el pulso. 2. ¿Es el dolor fuerte o leve? 3. ¿Ha comido hoy? 4. ¿Tiene alergia a algunas medicinas? 5. Señale dónde le duele. 6. ¿Tiene adormecida alguna parte del cuerpo? 7. ¿Tiene náusea?

Page 13

III. 1. Pain 2. Paramedic 3. Pulse 4. Blood pressure 5. Strong 6. Weak 7. Hospital 8. Allergies 9. Today 10. Here 11. Medicine 12. Consciousness 13. Nausea 14. Numbness 15. Fell 16. Body

Page 13

1. Fuerte 2. Hoy 3. Dolor 4. Paramédico 5. Pulso 6. Aquí 7. Leve 8. Conocimiento 9. Alergias 10. Hospital 11. Presión 12. Medicina 13. Cayó 14. Adormecida 15. Náusea

Page 13

1. Pulso, presión 2. Alergias 3. Dolor, leve 4. Hospital 5. Conocimiento

Page 14

1. When did it happen? 2. Today? 3. Where does it hurt? 4. Here? 5. What is the pain like? 6. Strong or weak? 7. Did you lose consciousness? 8. Did you eat today? 9. We're going to the hospital. 10. We're going to help. 11. I need to take your pulse. 12. I need to take your blood pressure. 13. Do you have allergies? 14. Do you have medicines? 15. Look up. 16. Do you have numbness in some part of the body? 17. Are you nauseated?

Pages 14-15

1. Necesito tomarle el pulso y la presión. 2. ¿Ha comido hoy? 3. ¿Dónde le duele? 4. ¿Es el dolor fuerte o leve? 5. ¿Perdió el conocimiento? 6. ¿Cuándo ocurrió? ¿hoy? 7. ¿Tiene alergias a alguna medicina? 8. Vamos a ayudar. 9. Vamos al hospital. 10. Cálmese. 11. No se preocupe. 12. Silencio, por favor. 13. Señale dónde le

duele. 14. ¿Tiene adormecida alguna parte del cuerpo? 15. ¿Tiene náusea?

Pages 15-16

1. Vamos a ayudar. Vamos al hospital. 2. Necesito tomar el pulso y la presión. Necesito ver la medicina. 3. ¿Tiene alergias a alguna medicina? 4. ¿Dónde le duele? 5. ¿Perdió el conocimiento?

Page 16

IV. 1. Señale dónde le duele. ¿Dónde le duele? 2. ¿Es el dolor fuerte o leve? ¿Cómo es el dolor? 3. ¿Cuándo ocurrió? 4. ¿Tiene alergias a alguna medicina? 5. ¿Perdió el conocimiento?

Chapter 3

Page 19

I. 1. Calm down. 2. Point. 3. Sit down. 4. Move. 5. Don't worry. 6. Lay down.

Page 19

1. Muévase. 2. Acuéstese en la camilla. 3. ¿Dónde está herido? 4. ¿Cuándo ocurrió? ¿Hace cuántas horas o minutos? 5. Necesito tomarle el pulso y la presión.

Page 21

III. 1. Hospital 2. Siéntese. 3. Muévase. 4. Gracias 5. Camilla 6. Herido 7. Horas 8. Minutos 9. Necesito 10. Silencio 11. Cuchillo 12. Pistola

Page 21

1. Señale dónde está herido. 2. Siéntese, por favor. 3. Cálmese. 4. Necesito tomarle el pulso y la presión. 5. Acuéstese en la camilla, por favor. 6. ¿Cuándo ocurrió? 7. Muévase, por favor. 8. No se preocupe. 9. ¿Dónde está el cuchillo? 10. Vamos al hospital.

Page 22

1. Silencio, muévase, por favor. 2. ¿Dónde le duele (está herido)? 3. Acuéstese en la camilla. 4. ¿Cuándo ocurrió? 5. Vamos al hospital. 6. No se preocupe.

Page 22

1. Cálmese. 2. Silencio. 3. Siéntese. 4. Acuéstese. 5.Muévase. 6. Señale.

Page 23

IV. 1. ¿Dónde está herido? 2. Acuéstese en la camilla. 3. Muévase, por favor.

Chapter 4

Page 26

I. 1. Help 2. Pain 3. Allergies 4. Medicines 5. Neck brace 6. Splint

Page 26

1. Alergias 2. Medicinas 3. Ayuda 4. Collar ortopédico 5. Tablilla 6. Dolor

Pages 26-27

1.¿Quién necesita ayuda? 2. Señale dónde le duele. 3. ¿Es el dolor fuerte, agudo, débil? ¿Se extiende el dolor? 4. No comprendo 5. ¿Tiene alergias a alguna medicina? 6. Necesito ponerle un collar ortopédico y una tablilla.

Page 29

III. 1. Questions 2. I need 3. Medicines 4. Prefer 5. Point/signal 6. Help 7. Allergies 8. Hospital 9. Pain 10. Silence 11. Neck brace 12. Strong 13. Weak/soft 14. Stretcher 15. Paramedic

Pages 29-30

1. No comprendo. 2. Señale dónde le duele. 3. ¿Es el dolor agudo? 4. ¿Es el dolor fuerte o leve? 5. Necesito ponerle un collar ortopédico. 6. Vamos a ponerle en la camilla. 7. ¿Toma medicinas? 8. ¿Qué hospital prefiere? 9. ¿Quién necesita ayuda? 10. ¿Tiene alergias?

Page 30

1. What? 2. Who?

Page 30

1. ¿Es el dolor fuerte o leve? 2. Tiene alergias a alguna medicina? 3. ¿Dónde le duele? 4. ¿Toma alguna medicina? 5. ¿Quién necesita ayuda? 6. ¿Qué hospital prefiere?

Pages 30-31

1. Más despacio. Cálmese, por favor. 2. ¿Quién necesita ayuda? 3. ¿Dónde le duele? ¿Dónde está herido? 4. ¿Cómo es el dolor? ¿Fuerte, leve, agudo? 5. ¿Qué medicina toma? 6. ¿Qué hospital prefiere? 7. Es necesario. 8. Vamos a ponerle una tablilla. 9. ¿Ha comido hoy?

Page 32

IV. 1. ¿Toma alguna medicinas? 2. ¿Dónde le duele? 3. ¿Tiene alergias a alguna medicina?

Chapter 5

Page 35

I. 1. Consciousness 2. Liquids 3. Illness 4. Stomach 5. Vomit 6. IV 7. Diarrhea 8. Chronic 9. Fever

Page 35

1. ¿Le duele el estómago? 2. ¿Perdió el conocimiento? 3. ¿Tiene vómitos o diarrea? 4. Vamos a ponerle un suero. No se preocupe.

Page 37

III. 1. ¿Qué le pasa? 2. ¿Le duele aquí? 3. ¿Tiene diarrea? 4. ¿Perdió el conocimiento? 5. ¿Ha bebido o comido algo hoy? 6. ¿Qué ha comido? 7. ¿Qué ha bebido?

Page 37

1. Necesito tomarle el pulso. 2. No se preocupe 3. Vamos a ponerle un suero. 4. No comprendo. 5. Necesita líquidos.

Pages 37-38

1. Necesito ponerle un suero. 2. Necesita liauidos. 3. ¿Le duele el estómago? 4. ¿Perdió el conocimiento? 5. ¿Tiene diarrea y vómitos?

Page 38

1. ¿Le duele el estómago? 2. ¿Tiene diarrea y vómitos? 3. Necesito ponerle un suero. 4. Necesito tomarle el pulso y la presión. 5. ¿Qué hospital prefiere?

Page 39

IV. 1. Acuéstese 2. ¿Cómo es el dolor? 3. ¿Cuándo? 4. ¿Cuándo?

Chapter 6

Page 42

I. 1. Para el corazón 2. Acuéstese 3. La medicina 4. Necesito 5. En la camilla 6. Náusea 7. Tiene 8. Señale 9. Dónde le duele

Page 42

1. El pulso y la presión 2. La camilla 3. Le duele 4. Náusea

Pages 43-44

III. 1. Lay down. 2. The stretcher 3. For 4. The heart 5. Here 6. Point 7. I need 8. We're going/Let's go 9. Where 10. "It" hurts me. 11. Take 12. The medicine 13. Paramedic 14. Well/good 15. To the hospital

Page 44

1. al hospital, vamos Vamos al hospital.
2. prefiere, que hospital ¿Qué hospital prefiere?
3. en la camilla, acuéstese Acuéstese en la camilla.
4. para el corazón, medicina, toma ¿Toma alguna medicina para el corazón?
5. hoy, la medicina, tomó ¿Tomó la medicina hoy?
6. náusea, tiene ¿Tiene náusea?

Pages 44-45

1. ¿Qué medicina toma? 2. ¿Dónde está la medicina? 3. ¿Dónde le duele? 4. ¿Tomó la medicina hoy? 5. Acuéstese en la camilla.

Page 45

IV 1. ¿Le duele el pecho? 2. ¿Dónde está la medicina? 3. ¿Toma digital? 4. ¿Qué hospital prefiere?

Chapter 7

Page 49

I. 1. Now 2. Before 3. Baby 4. Pain 5. Cesarean 6. Complications 7. Pregnant 8. Examine 9. "Water" fountain 10. Navel 11. Umbilical cord 12. It broke 13. Everything

Page 49

I. 1. ¿Está embarazada? 2. ¿Cuántos meses tiene de embarazo? 3. ¿Es su primer bebé? 4. Vamos a ayudarle. 5. No empuje, por favor.

Page 51

III. 1. Push 2. Male 3. Female 4. "Water" (fountain) 5. Baby 6. Tell me 7. Pains 8. First 9. Breathe 10. Slowly

Page 51

1. Are you about to give birth? 2. How many minutes apart are the pains? 3. Did your water break? 4. Did you have complications before? 5. How many months pregnant are you? 6. How many minutes apart are the pains (contractions)?

Page 52

1.¿Cuántos meses tiene de embarazo? 2. No se preocupe. Necesito examinarle. 3. Empuje, por favor. 4. Todo está bien. Es la placenta. 5. Es una hembra.

Page 52

1. ¿Está embarazada? 2. ¿Cuántos meses tiene embarazada? 3. ¿A cuántos minutos están los dolores? 4. ¿Es su primer bebé? 5. ¿Ya se le rompió la fuente? 6. ¿Tuvo complicaciones antes? 7. Por favor, empuje. 8. Respire lentamente. 9. Necesito cortar el cordón umbilical. 10. Es un varón.

Page 53

IV. 1. I don't know. 2. I want to push. 3. Oh, it really hurts! 4. The pain is starting. 5. It hurts a lot.

Page 54

1. Eight 2. Six 3. Five 4. Nine 5. Seven 6. Seven

Page 54

1. Five 2. Three 3. Two 4. Six 5. Four

Page 54

1. 5th 2. 8th 3. 4th 4. 6th 5. 2nd 6. 4th 7. 9th 8. 10th 9. 3rd 10. 7th

Pages 54-55

V. 1. ¿Está embarazada? 2. ¿Es su primer bebé? ¿Tuvo complicaciones antes? 3. Necesito examinarle. Todo está bien. 4. Por favor, respire lentamente y empuje. 5. Necesito cortar el cordón umbilical.

Index